RU Sept '16
05OCT21

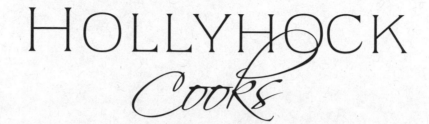

HOLLYHOCK
Cooks

food to nourish
body, mind
and soil

HOLLYHOCK
Cooks

*food to nourish
body, mind
and soil*

THE HOLLYHOCK COOKS *with*
Linda Solomon *and* Moreka Jolar

Photography by Maria Robledo

NEW SOCIETY PUBLISHERS
www.newsociety.com

Cataloguing in Publication Data:
A catalog record for this publication is available from the National Library of Canada.

Cover and book design by Diane McIntosh. Additional design and layout by Sue Custance and Greg Green.
Photographs by Maria Robledo.
Back cover photograph by Richard Truman.
Printed in Canada by Friesens.

New Society Publishers acknowledges the support of the Government of Canada through the Book Publishing Industry Development Program (BPIDP) for our publishing activities.

ISBN 13: 978-0-86571-488-5
ISBN 10: 0-86571-488-6

Inquiries regarding requests to reprint all or part of *Hollyhock Cooks* should be addressed to New Society Publishers at the address below.

To order directly from the publishers, please call toll-free (North America) 1-800-567-6772, or order online at www.newsociety.com
Any other inquiries can be directed by mail to:

New Society Publishers
P.O. Box 189, Gabriola Island, BC V0R 1X0, Canada
1-800-567-6772

New Society Publishers' mission is to publish books that contribute in fundamental ways to building an ecologically sustainable and just society, and to do so with the least possible impact on the environment, in a manner that models this vision. We are committed to doing this not just through education, but through action. We are acting on our commitment to the world's remaining ancient forests by phasing out our paper supply from ancient forests worldwide. This book is one step towards ending global deforestation and climate change. It is printed on acid-free paper that is **100% old growth forest-free** (100% post-consumer recycled), processed chlorine free, and printed with vegetable based, low VOC inks. For further information, or to browse our full list of books and purchase securely, visit our website at: www.newsociety.com

NEW SOCIETY PUBLISHERS   www.newsociety.com

Table of Contents

ONE: Salads and Dressings

TWO: Soups and Stews

THREE: Entrées

HOLLYHOCK *Cooks*

FOUR: On the Side

FIVE: Dips, Sauces and Pâtés

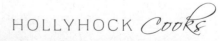

FIVE: Dips, Sauces and Pâtés *cont'd*

SIX: Baking

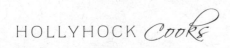

SEVEN: Desserts

EIGHT: Breakfast

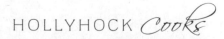

EIGHT: Breakfast *cont'd*

NINE: Drinks

Dedication

THIS BOOK IS DEDICATED TO EVERYONE who has ever worked in the Hollyhock kitchen and garden, and to the Hollyhock shareholders and board members for their support and vision. Your love and passion for good food have made this book possible.

Introduction

BODY, MIND AND SOIL are inextricably linked. It is in their interconnectedness that we find a root formula for global well-being.

The soil is where it all begins. Nutrition fuels human existence, and well-nourished humans are able to grow their minds. Intelligence, spirit, creativity, wisdom, accomplishment, compassion and love are the flowering of the human species.

Food is the first priority in human society. Our farming, manufacturing and distribution systems have grown in volume and standardization, and food has suffered alarming losses in nutrition and quality. The global-industrial food system is sacrificing the health of the natural world at a frightening rate. Soil is the ultimate source of planetary well-being. Treat it well and civilization thrives. Treat it badly and human existence is in peril.

Hollyhock supports humans learning to live a more healthy and balanced life, both as individuals and as citizens. Our work is to nurture and inspire those who are caring for the world. We bring people and organizations together to rest, learn, grow and strategize on behalf of community and society at large. We host outstanding teachers, businesses with social purpose and non-profits on the leading edge of social movements.

At the root of our work is love of the land, its care and its connection to the human spirit. We celebrate this relationship most visibly at our kitchen table, and our guests revel in the diverse and delicious globally influenced cuisine.

Cortes Island, our home, is famous for master gardeners and inventive cooks. Led by head chef, Debra Fontaine, our cooks are artists steeped in the British Columbian coastal temperate rainforest culture. So much is possible here due to the abundance of both land and sea. The long growing season, lush climate, and rich biodiversity combine to provide an enviable array of nutritious and organic options, as fresh and real as it gets.

The acclaimed and beloved Hollyhock "French intensive biodynamic" garden offers daily inspiration and ingredients to our guests and cooks. Heavenly teas, stunning floral arrangements, seeds for

At the root of our work is love of the land, its care and its connection to the human spirit.

HOLLYHOCK *Cooks*

1

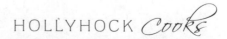

Sing the praises of real food prepared with love.

spreading far and wide, artworks, and contemplative reflection for the spirit, all grow robustly in our forest-meets-ocean soil.

Head gardener since the early 1980s, Nori Fletcher, has led a gifted team of devoted gardeners. Easy to imagine as temple monks, they go about double-digging, sowing, weeding, brewing compost, harvesting and pouring love into the soil and plants as a daily reminder to us all of the link between human body and mind, and the soil.

The British Columbian coast, our region, is internationally recognized and treasured as one of the planet's last great frontiers of nature. Hollyhock is famous for delectable and bountiful real food. The combination of the people and the natural world is our most important recipe.

We offer the recipes in this book as a current sampling of the delectable cuisine at Hollyhock. The miracle of memorable meals — using the freshest ingredients, learning from the satisfied tummy — is more than any scientific formula can capture. Seasonal rhythms, the type of soil, the variety, climactic shifts, and much more, make all good cooks artists. Only you, in your own kitchen, can know just the right touch of this or dollop of that needed to leave everyone longing for more.

We invite you inside the story of how Hollyhock cooks. We welcome your feedback about how the book works for you. Sing the praises of real food prepared with love. Celebrate the farmers whose lives are dedicated to the essential service of growing food. And please, make the extra effort to buy organic and local. Each effort is a contribution to the well-being of us all. We offer appreciation and praise to the many people who have been part of the Hollyhock kitchen and garden. Together we have grown Hollyhock as a living celebration of body, mind and soil.

— *Joel Solomon, Hollyhock Board Chair and*
Dana Bass Solomon, Hollyhock CEO

Welcome to Hollyhock

STEP OFF THE FERRY and take in the spectacular sight of the Coast Mountains and the coastal waters of the Georgia Strait. Your body relaxes, your mind expands and your psyche begins to shift as you absorb the vast beauty around you.

Everything intrusive and harsh from the fast world of cities and highways and North American consumer culture is left behind in a short journey. Weathered fishing boats line the dock, rocking on the gentle waves. Nearby a small island juts out of the water, rocky and green. Beyond it lies another island. In the water the translucent bodies of jellyfish drift with the currents. The air smells of cedar forests, sap and salty breeze.

One of the island's two taxis drives you up the road that is swathed in the green of Douglas firs. The combination of the exhilarating air and the stunning visual beauty practically puts you into a trance. Something has definitely shifted by the time you drive down Highfield Road and the taxi lets you out at Hollyhock. You register at the front desk, then enter a one-acre garden which explodes with flowers, fruit trees, herbs and vegetables.

It's as if you've walked into a van Gogh painting, the colors are so dramatic and the experience is so transcendent. The scents of the flowers, the soil and sea call you closer, making you want to breathe more deeply than you've wanted to do in a very long time. You follow the garden path to the gate and walk up towards the massage studio, venturing into the woods where huge ferns, ancient-looking cedars and towering pines line the trail. The earth in the woods feels soft beneath your feet. A huge yellow banana slug makes its way slowly across the path and you stoop down to study it. A deer bolts across the trail.

Later, inside the old farmhouse which is now the lodge, you pour yourself a glass of iced herbal tea and walk out onto the front deck where you sit down to enjoy the sight of the rocky beach. Starfish, oysters, clams, eels and crabs are exposed and then sheltered by the tide's eternal ebb and flow. You're eager to explore that rich coastal landscape, to take a dip in the ocean and then warm your body in the hot tub perched in a prime location for watching the sunset. A bald eagle flies across the sky and you watch in wonder. A gong rings, once, twice,

The combination of the exhilarating air and the stunning visual beauty practically puts you into a trance.

and once again, announcing dinner.

Back inside, the cooks stand behind the kitchen counter smiling as you look over the great feast prepared for tonight's meal. An array of colors, tastes, scents and sauces, a big bowl full of freshly picked lettuce dressed with edible orange nasturtium petals and bright yellow tulips await you. At the center of the table, a spectacular arrangement of white lilies and pink roses is a delightful adornment. Berries and cake on the kitchen counter make your mouth water. Welcome to Hollyhock. You've probably had to let go of a lot of busy-ness and stress to get here. Already it's worth it. This is going to be great, you think, filling your plate.

Hollyhock, Canada's leading educational retreat center, stands on the edge of the North American wilderness. Built several hundred feet above the high-tide line, Hollyhock provides a powerful space for people to converge and be nourished by pristine air, the lush rainforest and an ecstatic landscape of snow-capped mountains rising from the sea.

Is it a personal retreat center or a high-energy meeting facility? Sometimes it's hard to tell. When environmentalists, entrepreneurs, artists or intellectuals gather together to create closer community and hone their leadership skills, Hollyhock can seem like a dynamic conference center. When complete strangers convene to carve, dance, drum, sing, write, make paintings or masks, study mysticism or dreams, observe birds or make nature journals, do couples work, yoga or meditate, it can seem like the school we all wish we could have gone to from the very start.

Whoever is gathered at Hollyhock and whatever they're learning, one thing is certain — they're eating well. And guests at Hollyhock have eaten well for the last twenty years, since its founders put a down-payment on the old farmhouse, circular workshop buildings and living quarters that were the grounds of the 1970's experiential therapy center, the Cold Mountain Institute. They named it Hollyhock after the red hollyhocks growing at the edge of the garden. Ever since then Hollyhock's garden has supplied the kitchen with fresh vegetables, berries, herbs and flowers and provided homegrown organic ingredients for a dazzling array of primarily vegetarian entrées, breads, salads, and desserts cooked by many wonderful Hollyhock chefs.

ON CORTES ISLAND, to eat food is to understand good food, to love food, to grow food and to preserve food, no matter who you are or where you came from, or even whether you think of yourself as a cook. The need to get food, when the closest city is two hours away, to grow food in the high-producing summer months, to preserve food when the harvest comes in, and to cook it day after day, has produced some of North America's greatest domestic chefs.

Through all four seasons, local gardeners produce food that radiates life force, health and energy. In a community where take-out food is practically nonexistent, where pre-made food is extremely hard to find, and where the one coffee and cake shop, Trude's, opens only for short hours but to everyone's great delight, gastronomy depends on the natural resourcefulness of culinary genius that can only be cultivated with time and attention. Here on Cortes Island, the soil, the rocky shore and the sea offer up a natural feast.

The salmon boats are in. The farmer's markets are open. The gardens are bursting. Procuring wild fish fresh off the boat is one of the summer's greatest pleasures. Searching through the Linnea Farm vegetable stand and the farmers' market stalls for ingredients for tonight's dinner is another. Opening the prepared box of organic vegetables delivered weekly to your door by Blue Jay Lake forms a subtle link to urban centers like New York, San Francisco and Vancouver, where urban organic food deliveries provide an edible connection to rural life.

The best of Cortes Island cooking can be sampled at one of the island's many potluck dinners, where almost every guest brings a dish. Here you may find a talented master-carver roasting a freshly slain lamb over a fire. On the other side of the fire, a salmon fisherman has skewered his fresh catch and steams the clams he dug at sunset. Inside the house, salads full of freshly harvested winter fill hand-hewn wooden bowls on the counter. Beside the salads, sit braided breads baked with eggs from local chickens, and round European loaves prepared by a novelist, who composed a chapter in her mind while kneading the dough in her house by the sea. Then there are the

Here on Cortes Island, the soil, the rocky shore and the sea offer up a natural feast.

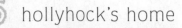

This rich local culture, culinary genius and the pristine natural environment provide ongoing inspiration for Hollyhock's cooks.

desserts, cooling in the corner where the children won't discover them until after dinner — cream puffs, fresh berry pies and delicious fluffy cakes.

The grill of the homemade barbecue balances over a circle of rocks by the beach. The fire toasts the mushrooms collected that afternoon by a former computer programmer, his rubber boots muddy from tromping deep into the woods with his basket of chanterelles, ceps and pine mushrooms. On the grill, the oysters sputtering in their gnarly shells are the same variety as the oysters which local oyster farmers export to Japan, New York City and nearby Vancouver. The delicious herbs brewing on the stove for tea come from the garden of the herbalist who cares for her flowers and healing plants as if they were a bevy of beloved children.

This rich local culture, culinary genius and the pristine natural environment provide ongoing inspiration for Hollyhock's cooks. They will continue to do so, as the ferries bring new and returning guests every season, and the tide comes in and the tide goes out.

May this book bring the taste of island elixir to you.

GOOD COOKING COMES FROM the same source as great art. Inspiration, together with determination and fresh organic ingredients, will transform the recipes you find here into world-class dishes and a fulfilling experience for you, the chef. The sight of a beautiful herb growing in the garden or popping out of the produce display can inspire a feast. The promise of a vegetable's summer succulence can move you to spend a few joyous hours in the kitchen.

What's on hand? What's fresh? These are the first questions to ask. That's the starting point for all the wonderful dishes that come out of the Hollyhock kitchen. If you can obtain organic produce and local or wild seafood, you're well on your way to making a fabulous dish. The fresher the produce, the better the dish. The more local the ingredients, the tastier they'll be.

Hollyhock is on a small island with only two general stores that carry a modest range of local organic produce, so what we can't grow in our own garden, we seek out in other local gardens. Local island growers produce fruits and vegetables that taste and look like nothing you'll ever find in the grocery store. We also support island fishers. All our fresh and smoked salmon is caught and smoked locally. Halibut and prawns come from local fishers. We will cook a meal according to what is available fresh at the dock. What we can't get on the island, we order in bulk from off the island. We're always altering the recipes we know to fit with what we have stored in the pantry and coolers.

The recipes you'll find here are representative of the vast array of food that comes out of the Hollyhock kitchen. We could have chosen any number of other combinations and variations, by any number of the talented and amazing cooks who pass through our kitchen. Hollyhock food is a continuously evolving cuisine that depends on the harvest of the garden and the passions of the cooks. This selection of recipes will give you the components you need to make many fabulous dishes. Once you've decided on a recipe, use it as a map and take detours. Substitute freely. We invite you to improvise, experiment and fall in love with cooking. Have fun. A cook who adores

The fresher the produce, the better the dish.

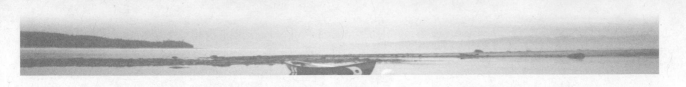

cooking will make dishes people love to eat. And although you might not succeed in getting it right every time, the more you turn to your own cabinets, local growers and unique tastes for inspiration, our recipes will become yours.

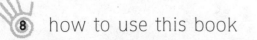

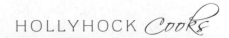

HOLLYHOCK *Cooks*

Blessing

All of you Gods there:
Our Mother-Parents-Father-Parents!
We, your flowers and sprouts
Who sprout at your feet and flower
In your arms
Sitting at your roots
And held in your branches,
We the eaters of food and the
Drinkers of liquid
Are further moved by your
Sustaining wombs and suckling
Breasts into a deeper entanglement
Of delicious spiritual debt
As you the great shimmering
Earth dazzles us into a forgetful ecstasy
In which we must
Remember how all things eat each other
To live in staggered moments
Of beauty only to feed another,
We the grateful amnesiacs
Today do not forget you
Do not throw you away as
You all the Holy animal and plant faces
Of the earth have never abandoned us
Please receive now a little bit of the
Magnificent aroma of the
Original Flowering Mountain Navel Earth

We remember you
Remembering us
Remembering you

Long Life
Honey in the heart
No Evil
Thirteen Thank yous.

— Food Blessing by Martin Prechtel, author of
Secrets of the Talking Jaguar and
Long Life, Honey in the Heart

ONE

Salads and Dressings

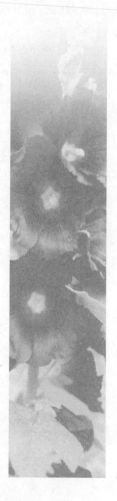

FOR YEARS GUESTS AT HOLLYHOCK have tried to convince the cooks to reveal the exact ingredients of the tangy yeast dressing that sits at the end of the buffet beside a large wooden salad bowl. At last it is time to reveal this and other secrets. Here you will find the herbs, spices and heavenly seasonings that account for the easy-to-make, wonderful-to-eat dressings that have caused so many Hollyhock guests to return to the salad bowl for seconds and thirds.

Lush beds of lettuce topped with brightly colored edible nasturtium petals make up the cornerstone of the Hollyhock lunch and dinner tables. Herbed dressings based on local raspberry vinegar, spicy Dijon mustard, tamari, or miso, lace the nutrient-rich lettuce harvested from the Hollyhock garden with elegant, complimentary tastes.

Because we don't have to ship it anywhere, our lettuce is more tender than most commercial varieties. The Hollyhock gardeners plant about 300 lettuce seedlings every two weeks for the spring, summer and fall. Good-tasting, delicate and colorful varieties of buttercrunch, romaine and looseleaf lettuce line different-sized hand-cultivated garden beds and a palate of greens and reds find their way from the garden into salads. We also cultivate many varieties of mixed greens such as arugula, endive, beet greens and kale, for added flavor. The fact that our lettuce is harvested and served within 24 hours accounts for its natural vitality and crunchy, delectable taste.

The Hollyhock cooks have made arranging refreshing and visually stunning salads a fine art. Recently harvested greens sprinkled with mild-tasting garden flowers like dahlias, hollyhocks, pansies and violas or nasturtiums are gorgeous to look at. And covering crisp lettuce with nuts, seeds, baked tofu, or bits of halibut turns a cool bed of organic greens into an intensely flavorful meal.

Salads adjust well to endless variations, so select the freshest vegetables at the market or from your garden and experiment with our mouth-watering recipes.

Asian Cucumber Salad

This is a refreshing, light and cooling salad. The cucumbers are spiced with the traditional Asian tastes of sesame, ginger and chili.

Serves 6-8

2	large long English cucumbers	2
⅓ cup	sesame oil	80 mL
⅓ cup	rice vinegar	80 mL
¼ cup	chopped fresh Thai basil or cilantro	60 mL
2 tbsp	grated fresh ginger	30 mL
½ tsp	salt	2.5 mL
½	seeded and minced jalapeño	½

1. Slice the cucumbers diagonally and thinly.

2. In a small bowl, whisk together the dressing ingredients. Dress the cucumbers immediately before serving. Garnish with sprigs of cilantro or Thai basil.

— *Moreka Jolar*

Asian Slaw

Thinly shredded Asian cabbage tossed with toasted peanuts and dressed in the classic Asian flavors of rice vinegar, ginger and chili make this a clean and refreshing side dish to any Asian meal. Toss in some shredded purple cabbage for bright color. It's a snap to prepare.

Serves 6-8

2 tbsp	sesame or peanut oil	30 mL
2 tbsp	rice vinegar	30 mL
1 tbsp	brown or white sugar	15 mL
1 tsp	grated fresh ginger	5 mL
	a pinch of chili flakes	
4 cups	shredded Asian cabbage such as su choy	960 mL
½ cup	dry-toasted peanuts	120 mL

1. In a small bowl, whisk together the oil, vinegar, sugar, ginger and chili flakes. Dress the cabbage with this dressing and toss it with the peanuts.

VARIATION
Use a spicy chili oil instead of the sesame or peanut oil if you prefer more heat.

— *Moreka Jolar*

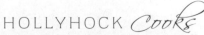

African Couscous Salad with Currants and Almonds

Couscous is a refined wheat and is known as the pasta of the Middle East. It is available in most groceries with specialty foods and is easy to prepare. Here couscous is combined with red and yellow bell peppers, sweetened with currants and cinnamon, sprinkled with slivered almonds to bring you intimations of North Africa, desert sands, and sun-drenched mountains. This salad is ideal for stuffing in pita pockets. Try adding green or yellow beans for variety.

1. Pour the boiling water over the couscous and the salt in a small bowl, cover and allow it to stand for 20 minutes, until you can fluff it with a fork.

2. Blanch the chopped carrots, peppers and onion by immersing them each in boiling water for a few minutes. Chill immediately.

3. In a small bowl, whisk together the dressing ingredients.

4. Combine the currants and almonds with the couscous and dressing. Add the vegetables and chill the salad before serving.

— *Linda Gardner*

Serves 6-8

1½ cups	dry couscous	360 mL
½ tsp	salt	2.5 mL
1¼ cups	boiling water	300 mL
1 cup	finely diced carrots	240 mL
1 cup	diced red and yellow bell peppers	240 mL
½ cup	finely diced purple onion	120 mL
½ cup	currants	120 mL
1 cup	toasted slivered almonds	240 mL

DRESSING

½ cup	olive oil	120 mL
¼ cup	lemon juice	60 mL
3 tbsp	chopped fresh parsley	45 mL
1 tbsp	chopped fresh mint	15 mL
½ tsp	salt	2.5 mL
½ tsp	ground cinnamon	2.5 mL

Carrot Salad with Lime

The taste is vibrant and clean, and the beets give the dish the vibrant hue of a West Coast sunset. The lime provides a tart zing to this healthy raw salad.

Serves 6-8

6 cups	shredded carrot	1.44 L
2	thinly diced red apples	2
½ cup	peeled and shredded beets	120 mL
I cup	toasted sunflower seeds	240 mL
¾ cup	freshly squeezed lime juice	180 mL
	salt to taste	

1. Combine all the ingredients and allow the mixture to chill for 1 hour before serving. Serve the salad in a bowl lined with whole cabbage leaves. If you like, add chopped fresh cilantro to taste.

— *Moreka Jolar*

Green Bean and Smoked Salmon Salad

Soil and sea converge in this beautiful green bean and salmon mélange that use Dijon mustard and purple onion to their greatest advantage. This fresh and tasty summer salad is quick, easy to make and most elegant.

Serves 6-8

8 cups	halved green beans	1.92 L
I tray	ice cubes, for chilling	I tray
⅓ cup	olive oil	80 mL
¼ cup	wine vinegar	60 mL
I tsp	prepared Dijon mustard	5 mL
7 oz.	flaked dry smoked salmon	200 g
2 cups	small cubed tomatoes	480 mL
I cup	finely diced purple onion	240 mL
2 tbsp	rinsed capers	30 mL
I tbsp	grated lemon zest	15 mL

1. Steam the green beans until they're bright green and tender. Transfer them immediately to a large bowl and toss them together with the ice cubes. This helps the beans to hold their vibrant color. When the beans are chilled, drain off the ice water.

2. In a small bowl, whisk together the oil, vinegar and Dijon mustard. Dress the beans with this dressing. Toss in the remaining ingredients and serve chilled.

— *Linda Gardner*

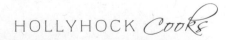

Green Bean Greek Salad with Macedonian-style Feta

Green beans, tomatoes, bell peppers and purple onion are combined with rich,
soft and creamy Macedonian-style feta to make this vibrant Greek salad.
Any other variety of feta can be used if preferred.

1. Steam the beans until tender, transfer them immediately to a bowl and toss them together with the ice cubes. This process of chilling helps the beans to keep their vibrant green color.

2. When the beans are chilled, strain off the ice and the water and combine the beans with the tomatoes, bell peppers and onion.

3. In a small bowl, whisk the dressing ingredients and toss with the salad. Serve garnished with crumbled feta and a wedge of lemon.

— *Moreka Jolar*

Serves 6-8

4 cups	halved green beans	960 mL
2 cups	tomatoes cut in large cubes	480 mL
2 cups	assorted bell peppers cut in large cubes	480 mL
1 cup	diced purple onion	240 mL
1 cup	crumbled Macedonian-style feta	240 mL
1 tray	ice cubes, for chilling	1 tray

DRESSING

3 tbsp	olive oil	45 mL
¼ cup	lemon juice	60 mL
1 tbsp	crushed garlic	15 mL
1 tbsp	chopped fresh basil	15 mL
1 tbsp	chopped fresh oregano	15 mL
1 tsp	black pepper	5 mL

" Hollyhock is a place that cultivates mindfulness, which is the art of being fully present. So when I come to the buffet line all my senses are open. The food is so beautiful and prepared with such love that it is a joy just to fill your plate. The colors, textures and smells are intoxicating. "
— *Joan Borysenko*

Halibut and White Bean Salad

You might stumble across this rustic salad in the hills of Tuscany. The salad is versatile and the flavor is mild and classic. It's a great way to turn last night's grilled fish into today's gourmet dish.

Serves 4-6

4 cups	cooked cannellini beans	960 mL
2 cups	cooked and flaked halibut	480 mL
4 tbsp	olive oil	60 mL
3 tbsp	fresh lemon juice	45 mL
3 tbsp	chopped fresh parsley	45 mL
4	thinly sliced scallions	4
	salt and pepper to taste	

1. Toss the beans and fish together in a large bowl.

2. In a small bowl, whisk together the remaining ingredients and dress the salad. Serve chilled next to a green salad or on its own.

VARIATIONS
You can use snapper or tuna or any other firm white fish instead of the halibut. Add a little fresh dill or some chipotle pepper for spice. Try adding 2 tablespoons of rinsed capers for a salty taste.

— Annie Rousseau

Mixed Vegetable Marinade Salad with Raspberry Vinaigrette

The sweet and exotic raspberry vinegar infuses the mixed steamed and fresh vegetables of this salad. Here is a salad that compliments a variety of entrées.

Serves 6-8

4 cups	broccoli cut in flowerets	960 mL
2 cups	cauliflower cut in flowerets	480 mL
2 cups	carrot cut in large cubes	480 mL
2 cups	red and yellow bell peppers cut in large cubes	480 mL
1 cup	cherry tomatoes sliced in half	240 mL
1 cup	slivered purple onion	240 mL
⅔ cup	raspberry vinegar *	160 mL
⅔ cup	extra virgin olive oil	160 mL
2 tsp	prepared Dijon mustard	10 mL
½ tsp	black pepper	2.5 mL
1 tbsp	chopped fresh chives	15 mL

1. Steam the broccoli, cauliflower and carrots in separate batches just until tender. The broccoli should steam for about 3-4 minutes and the cauliflower for 4-5 minutes. Combine the steamed vegetables in a medium-sized bowl and put immediately into the refrigerator to help retain their bright color. Add the peppers, tomatoes and onion.

2. In a small bowl, combine the raspberry vinegar, oil, Dijon mustard and pepper with a whisk and dress the salad. Toss in the chives. Allow the salad to chill and marinate for at least 2 hours before serving.

* Raspberry vinegar is an infusion of the sweet berries in vinegar. It is available in gourmet food shops or see page 120 for instructions on making your own.

— Moreka Jolar

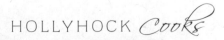

Salmon Salad with Capers and Chipotle

The smoked jalapeños or chipotle peppers make this salad stand out with its unique, bold flavor. Serve it chilled with crackers or in a pita, or sprinkle it over a green salad. It also makes an excellent sandwich filler.

1. In a medium-sized bowl, combine the salmon with the celery, bell peppers, scallions and capers.

2. In a small bowl, whisk together the vinegar, chipotle peppers and black pepper and dress the salmon salad. Season to taste with black pepper and garnish with capers.

* Small tins of chipotle peppers in adobo sauce are available in the Mexican foods sections of specialty food stores.

— *Moreka Jolar*

Serves 6-8

4 cups	cooked and flaked salmon	960 mL
I cup	finely diced celery	240 mL
I cup	diced red and yellow bell peppers	240 mL
4	chopped scallions	4
4 tbsp	red wine vinegar	60 mL
2 tsp	mashed chipotle peppers in adobo sauce *	10 mL
4 tbsp	rinsed capers	60 mL
I tsp	black pepper	5 mL

Orzo Salad with Smoked Salmon and Parsley Pesto

Orzo is a small, rice-shaped pasta and, chilled, makes an excellent base for savory salads. Here, the tender orzo pasta is tossed with sundried tomatoes, flakes of smoked salmon and dressed in a rustic parsley pesto.

Serves 6-8

1 lb.	orzo pasta	460 g
2 cups	Parsley and Pumpkin Seed Pesto (page 114)	480 mL
1 cup	sundried tomatoes	240 mL
5 oz.	flaked dry smoked salmon	145 g
2 cups	diced assorted bell peppers	480 mL
1 cup	diced purple onion	240 mL
¼ cup	rinsed capers	60 mL

1. If you are using dry sundried tomatoes and not those packed in oil, cover them with hot water and allow them to soak and soften for 30 minutes. Drain off the water and slice them thinly.

2. In a large pot, boil the orzo in a generous portion of water until tender. Drain and rinse in cold water.

3. Combine all the ingredients and serve on a bed of large lettuce leaves.

— *Moreka Jolar*

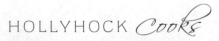

Pickled Arame Salad

Arame is a delicately flavored seaweed with a slightly sweet taste. Infused with vitality and rich oceanic minerals, this tasty seaweed salad can be served right after preparing, but is best when given a week to pickle. Serve it with an Asian dinner or savor it on its own.

1. Cover the dry arame generously with boiling water and allow it to stand for 1 hour, until the seaweed is soft. Drain. Add the sliced carrots and onions to the seaweed.

2. In a small bowl, combine 1 cup of water, rice vinegar, sugar and chili and whisk together until the sugar has dissolved. Add this to the seaweed.

3. Reserve the vinegar from the pickled ginger and add it to the seaweed with the ginger. Chill for at least 1 hour before serving. Garnish with chopped cilantro if desired.

— *Moreka Jolar*

Serves 4-6

2 cups	dry arame seaweed	480 mL
1 cup	very thinly sliced carrots	240 mL
½ cup	thinly sliced onion	120 mL
1½ cups	rice vinegar	360 mL
1 cup	water	240 mL
3 tbsp	sugar	45 mL
2 tsp	hot chili sauce or minced jalapeño	10 mL
¼ cup	thinly sliced pickled ginger	60 mL
½ cup	vinegar from the pickled ginger	120 mL

" Food is far more than sustenance. It provides some of the greatest pleasure in life. It connects us to other people: family, friends, community. It defines us culturally. "
— *Dr. Andrew Weil*

Sautéed Hijiki Salad

Hijiki is a rich, dark seaweed that radiates life force and means "bearer of wealth and beauty" in Japan where it has been used for hundreds of years. The dark strands of seaweed contrast beautifully with vibrant and crisp seasonal vegetables such as snow peas and carrots. This scrumptious salad makes an excellent accompaniment to oyster and fish dishes.

Serves 6-8

1 cup	dry hijiki seaweed	240 mL
1 tbsp	sesame oil	15 mL
¾ cup	diced onion	180 mL
1 tsp	minced garlic	5 mL
3 cups	thinly sliced seasonal vegetables such as snow peas, carrots, green or yellow beans, young yellow zucchini	720 mL
¼ cup	tamari or shoyu *	60 mL
	toasted sesame seeds to garnish	

1. Cover the dry hijiki with 2 cups (480 mL) of lukewarm water. Allow it to stand for 20 minutes. Drain.

2. In a large frying pan or wok, sauté the onion and garlic in a bit of sesame oil for a few minutes until the onion is transparent. Add the hijiki to the frying pan and continue to sauté for another 10 minutes.

3. Add the seasonal vegetables and tamari or shoyu and cook until the vegetables are tender. Garnish with toasted sesame seeds and serve warm or chilled, alone or over a bed of rice.

* Shoyu is a dark, rich and slightly sweet soy sauce and is available in Asian specialty food sections.

— *Martha Abelson*

"At Hollyhock it's all interconnected: the whole place is in harmony. The food is connected with the garden. The garden is connected with the teachings. The teachings are connected with the sky. The sky is connected with the water. Interconnected and inter-penetrated. That's why I teach at Hollyhock, because it's all one big united world up there."
— Natalie Goldberg

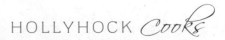

Spinach Salad with Crispy Apple and Toasted Cashews

Coat young spinach leaves with rich, creamy chèvre, then dress them up with lemon and garlic, and top it all off with tart apple slices and sweet toasted cashews. This is a wonderful salad — simple to prepare yet attractive and refined. It would not be out of place in a five-star restaurant.

1. Combine the dressing ingredients in a blender.
2. In a large bowl, crumble the goat's cheese over the spinach, toss and dress the salad right before serving. Top each serving with the toasted nuts and thinly sliced apples.

VARIATION
As an alternative to apples and cashews, you can use firm red Bartlett pears and chopped walnuts.

— *Moreka Jolar*

Serves 6-8

½ lb.	fresh young spinach leaves	230 g
6 oz.	chèvre — soft goat's cheese	170 g
2 cups	whole toasted cashews	480 mL
3	tart and crispy apples such as Granny Smith	3

DRESSING

¾ cup	olive oil	180 mL
⅓ cup	lemon juice	80 mL
1 tbsp	minced garlic	15 mL
1 tsp	salt	5 mL
½ tsp	pepper	2.5 mL
1 tbsp	honey	15 mL

Spinach Salad with Toasted Seeds

The toasted seeds add protein to this fresh, bold and crisp young spinach salad.
You can also sprinkle bit of grated Gouda cheese on top for extra taste.

Serves 6-8

½ lb.	fresh young spinach	230 g
3 cups	sliced fresh mushrooms	720 mL
1 cup	toasted pumpkin seeds	240 mL
½ cup	toasted sunflower seeds	120 mL
¼ cup	toasted sesame seeds	60 mL
1 cup	thinly sliced red bell pepper	240 mL

DRESSING

¾ cup	extra virgin olive oil	180 mL
¼ cup	white wine vinegar	60 mL
1 tbsp	honey	15 mL
2 tsp	crushed garlic	10 mL
2 tsp	prepared Dijon mustard	10 mL
1 tsp	mayonnaise	5 mL
	salt and pepper to taste	

1. Mix all the dressing ingredients together in blender or with a whisk.
2. In a salad bowl, toss the fresh spinach with the mushrooms, bell pepper and toasted seeds and bell pepper, reserving a few slices of the pepper for a garnish. Dress and serve immediately garnished with sliced bell peppers and, if you wish, some grated Gouda cheese.

— *Sylvie Rousseau*

cook's tip

The easiest way to toast seeds is to dry toast them in a skillet on low until they begin to brown. It also works to toast seeds on a baking sheet in the oven at 350°F.

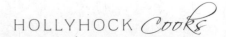

Purple Cabbage Slaw with Caraway and Currants

Thinly shredded carrots and vibrant purple cabbage are tossed with sweet currants and bold caraway seeds, then dressed in tangy yogurt to make this crisp and refreshing slaw.

1. Combine the cabbage and carrot in a medium-sized bowl.

2. In a small bowl, mix the yogurt with the vinegar, black pepper and caraway seeds and dress the slaw. Toss in the currants. Serve chilled.

— Moreka Jolar

Serves 6-8

2 cups	thinly shredded purple cabbage	480 mL
2 cups	shredded carrots	480 mL
1 cup	yogurt	240 mL
2 tbsp	red wine vinegar	30 mL
½ tsp	black pepper	2.5 mL
1 tbsp	whole caraway seeds	15 mL
¼ cup	currants	60 mL

Arugula, Pear and Romano Salad

Here is a tasty way to start off a pasta dinner. In this salad, the spicy tasting arugula is combined with salty Romano cheese and sweet pear. Use red Bartlett pears for a splash of sunset color in your salad.

1. In a large bowl, drizzle the oil and lemon juice over the greens and season with salt and pepper. Toss gently.

2. Arrange the salad on 6 salad plates and top each plate with slices of pear, cheese shavings and then sprinkle it with the chopped walnuts or hazelnuts. Serve immediately.

— Hanyu Wasyliw

Serves 6

6 cups	loosely packed arugula greens	1.44 L
3 tbsp	extra virgin olive oil	45 mL
1 tbsp	fresh lemon juice	15 mL
½ tsp	sea salt	2.5 mL
	black pepper to taste	
2	peeled, cored and sliced pears	2
3 oz.	coarsely grated or shaved Romano cheese	90 g
3 tbsp	toasted and coarsely chopped walnuts or hazelnuts	45 mL

Roasted Potato Salad with Chili Vinaigrette and Cilantro

This potato salad is richly textured but lower in fat than conventional potato salad.
Here is a new twist on an old favorite.

Serves 6

4-6 cups	potatoes cut in ½-inch cubes	1 - 1.5 L
¼ cup	olive oil	60 mL
1 cup	diced celery	240 mL
1 cup	red or yellow diced bell pepper	240 mL
5	sliced boiled eggs	5
1 cup	toasted and chopped walnuts	240 mL
½ cup	diced red onion	120 mL
2 tbsp	chopped cilantro	30 mL

DRESSING

3 tbsp	olive oil	45 mL
3 tbsp	rice vinegar	45 mL
2 tsp	crushed garlic	10 mL
1 tsp	salt	5 mL
1 tsp	mashed chipotle pepper in adobo sauce	5 mL

Preheat the oven to 400°F .

1. In a large bowl, toss the potatoes with the oil and roast them on a baking sheet in the oven at 400°F until they are tender and golden, about 30-45 minutes. Combine the cooled potatoes with the remaining salad ingredients in a bowl.

2. In a small bowl whisk together the dressing ingredients and dress the salad. Serve chilled.

— *Moreka Jolar*

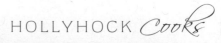

Yellow Beans with Honey Balsamic Vinaigrette and Oven-Roasted Cherry Tomatoes

What beautiful partners yellow beans and cherry tomatoes make. This salad is equally delicious hot or cold. Crumble a bit of soft goat's cheese or feta on top to create a richer and creamier dish.

Preheat the oven to 400°F.

1. Toss the cherry tomatoes with the garlic, 3 tbsp of the olive oil and the black pepper. Roast the tomatoes in a casserole dish in the oven for 25-30 minutes, stirring occasionally.

2. Steam the beans just until they are tender.

3. In a small bowl, whisk together the vinegar, the remaining 2 tbsp of olive oil, basil and honey and pour over the warm beans. Place on a serving platter. Arrange the warm cherry tomatoes over the beans and serve immediately.

— *Moreka Jolar*

Serves 8-10

6 cups	whole cherry tomatoes	1.44 L
1 tbsp	crushed garlic	15 mL
5 tbsp	olive oil	75 mL
1 tsp	black pepper	5 mL
8 cups	yellow beans, snapped in half	1.92 L
¼ cup	balsamic vinegar	60 mL
2 tbsp	chopped fresh basil	30 mL
1 tbsp	honey	15 mL

Tofu Salad

This protein-rich alternative to egg salad can stand on its own or be used to fill pita bread and sandwiches. It's best when allowed to chill in the refrigerator for at least two hours before serving.

Serves 2-4

I lb.	crumbled soft tofu	460 g
½ cup	diced red bell pepper	120 mL
½ cup	diced celery	120 mL
2 tbsp	chopped fresh parsley	30 mL
2 tbsp	finely diced onion or scallions	30 mL
2 tbsp	regular or tofu mayonnaise (page 119)	30 mL
2 tsp	Spike * or salt	10 mL
½ tsp	curry powder	2.5 mL
½ tsp	turmeric	2.5 mL

1. In a medium-sized bowl, combine all the ingredients thoroughly. Be careful to keep some of the texture of the tofu. Chill for at least 2 hours before serving.

* Spike is sea salt seasoned with vegetables.

— *Moreka Jolar*

 cook's tip

Always store tofu in the fridge, covered generously with water. Changing the water every few days will help to keep it fresh.

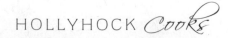

Tabouleh with Toasted Seeds

This nutritious Middle Eastern salad is oil-free and can keep you cool on the hottest summer day. Bulgur wheat is the cornerstone, but the lemon juice and herbs give this salad a light and refreshing taste.

1. In a medium-sized bowl, combine the bulgur wheat with the salt and garlic and add the boiling water. Cover it with plastic wrap or a tight lid and allow it to stand for 30-40 minutes. Remove the lid, fluff the cooked bulgur wheat with a fork and chill.

2. In a large bowl, toss the chilled bulgur with the remaining ingredients and serve immediately.

— *Moreka Jolar*

Serves 6-8

1 cup	bulgur wheat	240 mL
1 tbsp	crushed garlic	15 mL
1 tsp	salt	5 mL
2 cups	boiling water	480 mL
2 cups	cubed cucumber	480 mL
1 cup	finely diced purple onion	240 mL
1 cup	diced red and yellow bell peppers	240 mL
1 cup	chopped fresh tomatoes	240 mL
1 cup	packed chopped fresh parsley	240 mL
	juice of 2 lemons	
1 cup	whole toasted sunflower, pumpkin or sesame seeds	240 mL
	salt and pepper to taste	

Green Goddess Dressing

This is the ultimate spring and summer dressing. Versatile, thick, creamy and bright green in color, this dressing brings all the bold flavors of your favorite herbs to the table. Serve it over fresh or steamed greens or vegetables and enjoy.

Makes 4 cups

2 cups	packed fresh herbs *	480 mL
1½ cups	apple cider vinegar	360 mL
1 cup	water	240 mL
½ cup	miso paste	120 mL
1	seeded and minced jalapeño	1
1 tbsp	crushed garlic	15 mL
1 cup	sunflower or safflower oil	240 mL

1. In a blender, combine the herbs, vinegar and water thoroughly, mixing for about a minute on high. While mixing, add the miso, jalapeño and garlic, and process for another 30 seconds. Then begin to drizzle in the oil while still mixing. Stop blending as soon as all the oil has been added. The dressing will be thick and creamy.

2. Keep refrigerated. Allow the dressing to warm slightly at room temperature before serving. The dressing will keep for up to 2 weeks.

* Choose herbs such as parsley and basil with smaller bits of other stronger herbs such as oregano, dill, thyme, cilantro, chives, and rosemary.

— *Moreka Jolar*

 cook's tip

Do not underestimate the heat of a jalapeño. To avoid "pepper burn," wear latex gloves or coat your hands in oil before mincing this spicy pepper.

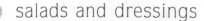

 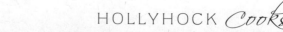

Hollyhock Yeast Dressing

Here it is — the long-awaited secret of Hollyhock's most popular salad dressing.
Dark and intensely flavored, this dressing is versatile and rich in B vitamins.
It's tastes delicious on cooked grains as well as on fresh greens.

1. Combine the first 5 ingredients in a blender until they are thoroughly mixed. While still mixing on high, pour the oil in a slow, steady stream. Add all the oil or stop when a desired consistency is reached. When refrigerated this dressing will keep for up to 2 weeks.

* Nutritional flake yeast comes from molasses (it grows on molasses) and is rich in B vitamins. It is available in natural food stores. Do not confuse it with brewer's yeast, its darker and powdered cousin.

Makes 2½ cups

½ cup	nutritional flake yeast *	120 mL
⅓ cup	water	80 mL
⅓ cup	soy sauce or tamari	80 mL
⅓ cup	apple cider vinegar	80 mL
2 tbsp	crushed garlic	30 mL
1½ cups	sunflower oil	360 mL

— *Moreka Jolar*

Hollyhock Creamy Herbal Dressing

The raspberry vinegar in this dressing creates a delightful pink blush and delicate flavor. If you have no raspberry vinegar on hand, mash up a handful of fresh raspberries and whisk them in. Lace this dressing over steamed vegetables, new potatoes, kale or rice.

Makes 2½ cups

1 cup	yogurt	240 mL
½ cup	buttermilk	120 mL
½ cup	mayonnaise	120 mL
¼ cup	finely chopped fresh parsley	60 mL
¼ cup	finely chopped fresh chives	60 mL
1 tbsp	finely chopped fresh dill	15 mL
2 tbsp	raspberry vinegar * or cider vinegar	30 mL
½ tsp	salt	2.5 mL
¼ tsp	black pepper	1.2 mL
	a dash of hot sauce to taste	

1. Combine all the ingredients with a whisk. Keeps refrigerated for up to 1 week.

* Raspberry vinegar is available in specialty delis or see page 129 for instructions on making your own.

— *Moreka Jolar*

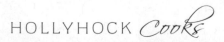

Hollyhock Poppyseed Dressing

This Hollyhock standard is slightly sweet and spicy in taste. Poppyseeds provide the subtle crunch and give an appealing aesthetic to this lovely salad dressing.

1. In a blender, process all the ingredients except the poppyseeds and oil for 30 seconds, until they are well combined. While still blending on high, add the poppyseeds and then add the oil gradually and in a steady stream. Stop blending as soon as all the oil has been added. This dressing keeps refrigerated for up to 2 weeks.

Makes 2½ cups

½ cup	water	120 mL
¼ cup	cider vinegar	60 mL
¼ cup	diced onion	60 mL
2 tbsp	honey	30 mL
2 tbsp	prepared Dijon mustard	10 mL
2 tsp	salt	30 mL
1 tbsp	poppyseeds	15 mL
1½ cups	sunflower or safflower oil	360 mL

Sesame Maple Dressing

Sweet and with a strong aroma of sesame, this dressing can be served over green salads or steamed Asian greens. It makes a scrumptious fish marinade, too.

1. Mix everything except the oils in a blender. Combine the 2 oils and slowly add to blender while mixing. Stop mixing as soon as all the oil has been added.

— *Moreka Jolar*

Makes 1½ cups

⅓ cup	tamari	80 mL
¼ cup	water	60 mL
¼ cup	maple syrup	60 mL
2 tsp	prepared Dijon mustard	10 mL
1 tsp	minced garlic	5 mL
⅓ cup	sunflower or safflower oil	80 mL
3 tbsp	sesame oil	45 mL

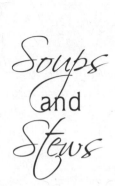

TWO

Soups and Stews

IT'S THE SEASONING the makes the soup at Hollyhock, where we benefit from a selection of herbs harvested fresh daily. Hand-picked, lovingly tended and carefully selected culinary herbs, such as French tarragon, parsley, sweet basil, Thai basil, Greek oregano, cilantro, chives, dill leaves and flowers, thyme, rosemary, mint and French sorrel fill Hollyhock soups and stews, infusing them with various flavors. In the peak of our growing season, the gardeners harvest 192 bunches of these aromatic taste enhancers.

In the summer, herbs are dried and put aside to use in soups and stews in the fall and spring. Soups offer a great way to bring out the full flavor of an herb. Making broth from fish or vegetables and keeping it on hand in the freezer to be thawed on demand is an efficient way to turn out savory brews with the simple addition of choice vegetables. Vegetables of contrasting colors create eye-pleasing soups and stews. Adding legumes yields a heartier mixture.

Many soups and stews taste better the day after they are cooked, when the vegetables and herbs have had a chance to thoroughly permeate the broth with their fusion of tastes. Make a big enough batch to eat some now and have a batch to freeze and bring out later when you need a quick and easy meal. Blending the ingredients creates creamier, smoother textures.

At Hollyhock, we cook according to the feeling of the day. On a hot summer day, we serve a light soup such as Fresh Green Soup (page 39). On a chilly day, we serve a spicy, warming stew or soup such as Prawn and Snapper Stew (page 42).

Soup reflects the unique flavors of a culture. Tumeric and cumin give Dal (page 36) its Indian taste. Chipotle peppers in adobo sauce turn black bean soup (page 34) into a distinctly Mexican dish. Hot pimento paste makes a unique fish stew (page 45) defined by its fiery spice. A base of coconut milk spiced with red curry paste, lemon grass and lime leaves calls up the fusion of hot and cool sensations that could only be Thai (page 44).

Soups and stews are at the center of many delicious Hollyhock lunches and reflect the fusion of global and local culture. Locally grown produce and globally inspired recipes spiced with fresh herbs make the following selection of soups and stews exciting, nutritious and delicious.

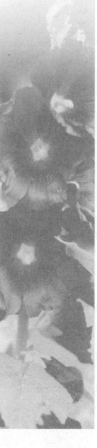

Black Bean Soup with Chipotle and Orange

Topped with a spoonful of sour cream or yogurt, this thick soup with a subtle orange flavor will provide warmth on a cold night. Serve with Best Ever Cornbread (page 124) or Savory Zucchini Muffins (page 144) and a salad for a delicious and nutritious lunch or supper.

Serves 6-8

2 tbsp	sunflower or safflower oil	30 mL
2 cups	chopped onion	480 mL
2 cups	finely diced carrot	480 mL
1 tbsp	minced garlic	15 mL
1 tsp	salt	5 mL
2 tsp	mashed chipotle peppers in adobo sauce *	10 mL.
2 tsp	ground cumin	10 mL
4 cups	cooked black beans	960 mL
4 cups	water	960 mL
3 cups	chopped fresh tomato	720 mL
1 cup	freshly squeezed orange juice	240 mL

1. In a large soup pot, sauté the onion, carrots and garlic in the oil for about 5 minutes. Add the salt, chipotle peppers and cumin and continue to cook and stir for another 5 minutes. Add the black beans and water, cover and simmer for 30 minutes.

2. Process half of the cooked soup in a blender or with a hand-held processor and add it back to the soup pot. Add the chopped tomato and orange juice and gently reheat before serving.

* Chipotle peppers in adobo sauce are available in small tins in groceries with a Mexican food's section.

— *Moreka Jolar*

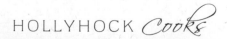

Borscht

On Cortes Island, organically grown beets are sweet and delectable and borscht comes in many different ways. Garnished with yogurt or sour cream and chives, this recipe is a local favorite, loved even more when served with Caraway Rye Bread (page 126) and Tofu Salad (page 26).

1. In a large soup pot, sauté the onion, garlic and bay leaves in oil until tender. Add the cubed beets and continue to sauté, for approximately 20 minutes, just until beets begin to get tender. Add the carrots, cabbage and tomatoes and the water or vegetable stock. Cover and simmer until the beets and carrots are completely tender, about 45 minutes to an hour.

2. Remove any foam that may have formed on the surface. Season with salt and lots of pepper to taste. Stir in the fresh dill and serve hot, garnished with sour cream or yogurt.

— *Moreka Jolar*

Serves 6-8

2 tbsp	sunflower or safflower oil	30 mL
2 cups	chopped yellow onion	480 mL
2 tsp	crushed garlic	30 mL
2	bay leaves	2
6 cups	peeled beets cut in ¼ inch-cubes	1.44 L
1 cup	diced carrot	240 mL
½	large purple cabbage, shredded	½
3 cups	chopped fresh tomatoes	720 mL
6-8 cups	water or vegetable stock	1.4 - 2 L
	salt and pepper to taste	
¼ cup	chopped fresh dill	60 mL
	yogurt or sour cream to garnish	

Dal

A must at an Indian meal, protein-rich dal tastes delicious over rice or served on its own.
To fill it out and make a stew, add two cups of chopped fresh tomatoes and three
cups of packed chard or spinach and heat until the greens are wilted.

Serves 3-5

2 cups	dry red lentils or yellow mung beans	480 mL
5 cups	water	1.2 L
2 tsp	turmeric	10 mL
1 tsp	salt	5 mL
2 tsp	whole cumin seeds	10 mL
2 tbsp	butter or oil	30 mL
1 cup	finely diced onion	240 mL
1½ tbsp	crushed garlic	8 mL
1 tbsp	grated fresh ginger	15 mL
2 tsp	whole black mustard seeds	10 mL
1 cup	coconut milk	240 mL

1. Rinse and check the lentils or mung beans for stones before putting them in a heavy saucepan with water, turmeric and salt. Bring to a boil and then simmer for approximately 30-40 minutes, until the lentils or beans turn very soft and mushy. Stir often to avoid sticking.

2. In medium-sized frying pan, dry toast the cumin seeds until they begin to turn brown. Allow them to cool before grinding the seeds in a coffee or spice grinder.

3. In the same frying pan, sauté the onion, garlic, ginger and whole mustard seeds in a bit of butter or oil until the onion is transparent. Add the ground cumin to the frying pan, combine well and then add to the cooked lentils or beans. Continue to simmer for another 15 minutes, reduce the heat and stir in the coconut milk. Serve hot.

— *Rowan Brooks*

cook's tip

Store whole fresh ginger in the freezer. When you are ready to use a bit, it is easy to peel and grate while still frozen and frezing it minimizes those nasty ginger hairs. Place the remaining ginger back in the freezer.

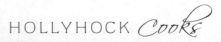

HOLLYHOCK *Cooks*

Carrot Soup with Tahini

Tahini, ginger and cumin coalesce in this delectable blended, silky carrot soup.
Serve it with Honey Curry Bread (page 132) or Roulade with Green Olive
Tapenade (page 109) for a vitamin-A-rich feast.

1. In a medium-sized soup pot, sauté the onion, ginger, garlic, cumin seeds
   and chili flakes in the oil until the onion is transparent, approximately
   15 minutes. Add the carrots and continue to sauté for another
   10 minutes. Add the water or stock and then cover and allow it to
   boil for 45 minutes, or until the carrots are tender.

2. Transfer half of the soup to a blender or food processor. Mix it on low
   for about 10 seconds and put it back in the soup pot.

3. Stir in the tahini and basil, salt to taste and serve immediately. Reheat
   slightly, if necessary, but do not boil it or the tahini will separate.

— *Moreka Jolar*

Serves 6-8

2 tbsp	sunflower or safflower oil	30 mL
2 cups	diced onion	480 mL
1 tbsp	minced fresh ginger	15 mL
2 tsp	crushed garlic	10 mL
1 tsp	whole cumin seed	5 mL
½ tsp	red chili flakes	2.5 mL
6 cups	coarsely chopped carrots	1.4 L
8 cups	water or stock	1.9 L
½ cup	tahini	120 mL
1 tbsp	chopped fresh basil	15 mL
	salt to taste	

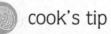 cook's tip

*Be careful of hot liquid in blenders.
It tends to explode out of the top. It's best
to remove the small cap of the blender lid
and hold down several layers of tea towel
on it while you blend on low speed.
Under-fill the blender. Mixing a half a
blender full of hot soup at a time is the
safest way.*

Chilled Avocado Soup

This soup is made for the shade on a scorching summer day.
It is delightfully, rich and oh, so elegantly cool.

6 small servings

5	soft ripe avocados, or 3-4 cup mashed	5
⅓ cup	fresh lime juice	80 mL
⅔ cups	chopped fresh tomatoes	.5 - .75L
1½ cups	chilled vegetable soup stock or broth	360 mL
3 tbsp	chopped fresh cilantro	45 mL
1-2 tsp	chili sauce such as Tabasco sauce	5 - 10mL
	salt to taste	
3	small corn tortillas	3
4 tbsp	sunflower or safflower oil	60 mL

1. Process the avocado and lime juice in a food processor until smooth. Transfer this mixture to a large bowl and add the chopped tomatoes, soup stock, coriander and chili sauce. Season with salt to taste. Cover with plastic and refrigerate for 1 hour.

2. Meanwhile, cut the tortillas into thin, ¼-inch strips and shallow fry them in oil until golden and crisp. Allow them to drain on a paper towel.

3. Serve the soup chilled and garnished with crispy tortilla strips. If you like, you can also garnish the soup with a spoonful of sour cream and more chopped cilantro.

— *Linda Gardner*

Pear and Parsnip Soup

This soup has a hint of nutmeg and is delicate and light in flavor. It improves in taste when refrigerated overnight and served the next day. It is also nice served with granary buns and spinach salad with toasted seeds.

Serves 6-8

2 tbsp	sunflower or safflower oil	30 mL
2	chopped onions	2
5-6	peeled and grated parsnips	5-6
6-8 cups	vegetable stock or water	1.5 - 2 L
3 cups	peeled and chopped fresh pears	720 mL
2 tsp	chopped fresh thyme	10 mL
	pinch of nutmeg	
	salt and pepper to taste	
	yogurt to garnish	

1. In a soup pot, sauté the onions in the oil for 2 minutes. Add the parsnips and cook for another 3 minutes, stirring constantly.

2. Add the stock or water, pears, thyme and nutmeg. Bring it to a boil and simmer for 10-15 minutes or until the pears are tender.

3. Process all the soup in a blender or serve it as is. Season with salt and pepper to taste. Garnish with yogurt. Serve hot.

— *Annie Rousseau*

Fresh Green Soup

This soup contains the smooth and delicate taste of summer herbs. It is great for those who have a large zucchini patch. Serve it with Spicy Cornmeal Muffins (page 146).

1. In a large soup pot, sauté the onion and celery in the oil until soft.

2. Rinse the split peas. Add 4 cups of the vegetable stock or water, the split peas and the bay leaf to the soup pot with the onions and celery. Bring the mixture to a boil and then cover and simmer on low heat for approximately 40 minutes.

3. Add the zucchini and remaining stock or water. Cook for another 15 minutes or until the zucchini is soft. Remove the bay leaf and purée the soup in a blender. Return the puréed ingredients to the soup pot and stir in the spinach or chard, parsley and basil. Season with salt and pepper to taste and cook just until the greens have wilted. Serve hot.

— Annie Rousseau

Serves 6-8

2 tbsp	sunflower or safflower oil	30 mL
I cup	chopped onion	240 mL
2 cups	diced celery	480 mL
6 cups	stock or water	1.4 L
¾ cup	dry green split peas	180 mL
I	bay leaf	I
6 cups	diced zucchini	1.4 L
8-10 cups	packed fresh spinach or chard, washed and chopped	2 - 2.5 L
¼ cup	chopped fresh parsley	60 mL
2 tsp	chopped fresh basil	10 mL
	salt and pepper to taste	

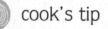 cook's tip

Vegetable stock is a great thing to have around. As you cook your meal, throw all the ends of vegetables that you would normally compost such as onions, carrots, celery etc. into a large pot of water on the stove. Add a couple bay leaves, a bunch of parsley and other fresh herbs. Allow this pot to boil all afternoon, strain off the vegetables and reserve the stock for a soup base. This will freeze well. Avoid strongly flavored and brightly colored vegetables such as beets, broccoli, cabbage, asparagus and fennel.

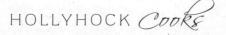

Mixed Bean Chili with Corn

Put this chunky chili over brown rice for a protein-rich meal or serve it on its own.
Ancho chili gives the soup a rich flavor but is not known for its spicy heat, so add
chili pepper for more kick. Stir in some grated cheddar, fresh cilantro or crumbled tofu,
if desired, and serve it with our Best Ever Cornbread (page 124).

8-10 servings

2 tbsp	sunflower or safflower oil	30 mL
2 cups	coarsely chopped onion	480 mL
2 cups	coarsely chopped carrot	480 mL
1 tbsp	crushed garlic	15 mL
1 cup	chopped celery	240 mL
2 tbsp	ancho chili powder	30 mL
1½ tsp	salt	7.5 mL
1½ tsp	paprika	7.5 mL
4 cups	various cooked and combined beans, such as kidney, pinto or black beans	960 mL
2 cups	coarsely chopped yellow zucchini	480 mL
2 cups	coarsely chopped bell peppers	480 mL
6-8 cups	coarsely chopped fresh tomatoes	1.5 - 2 L
2 cups	corn kernels, fresh off the cob or frozen	480 mL

1. In a large soup pot, sauté the onions, carrots and garlic in the oil for 10-15 minutes. Add the celery, ancho chili powder, salt and paprika and continue to sauté for 5 minutes. Add the beans, zucchini, bell peppers, and tomatoes. Cover and simmer for 30-45 minutes or until all the vegetables are tender, stirring every 10 minutes to stop it from sticking.

2. Just before serving, stir in the corn and continue to simmer for 5 minutes. Serve hot.

— Moreka Jolar

cook's tip

It's cheaper and better for the environment to avoid using canned beans. Dry beans taste better and will store for a long time. Allow them to soak overnight, topped generously with water. The next day, drain the water and refill with fresh water and then cook. Adding a couple of bay leaves and a handful of coriander seeds helps to make beans easier to digest.

Portuguese Potato and Kale Soup

Potatoes come in a remarkable variety of shapes, sizes and colors. Ask your local grower for their favorite color and variety of this wonderful vegetable, brought to North America originally from the Andes Mountains. Kale thrives on Cortes Island all through the fall and the winter and it shows up in the most interesting dishes, like this delicious soup with its proud European overtones. Drizzle olive oil over the top.

1. In a heavy-bottomed soup pot, sauté the onions in the olive oil until soft, approximately 4-5 minutes. Add the garlic and sauté for another minute, stirring constantly. Add the salt, water or stock and diced potatoes. Bring the soup to a boil.

2. Reduce the heat and simmer, stirring occasionally, until the potatoes fall apart. This will take about 1 hour. Mash any remaining large chunks of potato with a potato masher or a large spoon until you have a coarse purée.

3. Add the shredded kale and let it simmer for another 5 minutes or so, until the kale is tender but still bright green. Season with pepper to taste.

— *Hanyu Wasyliw*

Serves 6

3 cups	diced onions	720 mL
2 tsp	minced garlic	10 mL
¼ cup	olive oil	60 mL
2 tsp	salt	10 mL
8-10 cups	water or vegetable stock	2 - 2.5 L
5 cups	peeled and diced potatoes	1.2 L
2 cups	finely shredded kale leaves or packed collard greens	480 mL
	black pepper to taste	

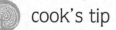 cook's tip

Cooking time for the potatoes varies according to the type of the potato used. Russet or baking potatoes will cook the fastest.

Prawn and Snapper Stew with Leeks and White Wine

Delicate in flavor, this classic seafood stew is a chunky and filling meal on its own.
It is also delightful with Savory Zucchini Muffins (page 144) or Pissaladière (page 139).
Other white fish, such as cod or halibut, can stand in for the snapper.

Serves 6-8

4 cups	leeks cut into thin rounds	960 mL
1 tbsp	butter	15 mL
3 cups	new potatoes cut in small cubes	720 mL
½ tsp	fresh thyme	2.5 mL
½ tsp	chopped fresh marjoram	2.5 mL
½ tsp	black pepper	2.5 mL
5 cups	water or seafood stock	1.2 L
2 cups	diced yellow bell peppers	480 mL
2 cups	diced roma tomatoes	480 mL
1 lb.	snapper fillet	460 g
1 lb.	shelled prawn tails	460 g
¼ cup	dry white wine	60 mL
	salt to taste	

1. In a large soup pot, sauté the leeks in the butter until they become tender. Add the potatoes, thyme, marjoram and pepper and sauté them for another 10 minutes. Add the water, or stock, bell peppers, and tomatoes to the pot. Cover and simmer for 15 minutes.

2. Cut the snapper with a sharp knife into 1-inch cubes. Use strong tweezers or small pliers to pull out any stray bones in the snapper without tearing this delicate fish.

3. Add the prawn tails, snapper pieces and wine and simmer uncovered for 2 minutes or just until the fish is white and flaky. Serve immediately.

— *Moreka Jolar*

cook's tip

Prawn shells make great stock for seafood stews. Boil the shells in a generous amount of water for one hour, strain off the shells and reserve stock. This will freeze well for up to one month.

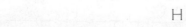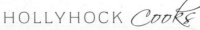

Spicy Squash Soup with Roasted Garlic and Yogurt

This is a spicy, ethnic and creamy soup, with a fusion of classic Indian spice, sweet roasted garlic and squash. A flair of vindaloo curry paste turns this squash extravaganza into a tasty little feast.

1. In a large soup pot, sauté the onion, curry paste and pepper in a bit of butter or oil until the onion is just beginning to brown. Add the ginger, squash and water and whole garlic cloves. Cover and simmer until the squash is very tender, approximately 30-45 minutes.

2. Mash the soup with a potato masher or purée it until it begins to be smooth. Add the yogurt and gently reheat but don't let it boil.

* Vindaloo curry paste is available in groceries with an Indian foods section.

— *Kaeli Robinsong*

Serves 6-8

2 cups	chopped onion	480 mL
1 tsp	vindaloo curry paste *	5 mL
1 tsp	black pepper	5 mL
3 tbsp	grated fresh ginger	45 mL
6 cups	peeled and cubed acorn, delicata, or butternut squash	1.4 L
7 cups	water or stock	1.7 L
8	whole cloves of roasted garlic	8
2 cups	yogurt	480 mL
	salt to taste	

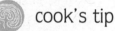 cook's tip

To roast garlic cloves, toss them in a bit of oil and roast them in a frying pan or on baking sheet in a 400° F oven until the garlic begins to turn brown on all sides.

 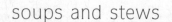

Thai Sweet Potato Soup

Cilantro, lemongrass, coconut milk and peanuts make this easy-to-prepare and lightly spiced soup an explosion of flavor.

6-8 Servings

2 cups	chopped onion	480 mL
1 tsp	crushed garlic	5 mL
2	lime leaves *	2
2 tsp	Thai red curry paste *	10 mL
6 cups	peeled and cubed sweet potatoes	1.4 L
7 cups	water or stock	1.7 L
1 stick	lemongrass	1 stick
¼ tbsp	crunchy peanut butter	4 mL
2 cups	coconut milk	480 mL
	salt to taste	
	a little bunch of fresh cilantro	

1. In a large soup pot, sauté the onion, garlic and lime leaves for 10 minutes.

2. Pound the lemongrass with a rolling pin until it looks bruised.

3. Add the curry paste and cook 1 minute before adding the sweet potatoes, water or stock, lemongrass and peanut butter. Cover and simmer the soup for 30-45 minutes or until the sweet potato is soft.

4. Remove the lime leaves and lemongrass and mash or purée the soup.

5. Add the coconut milk and season with salt to taste. Gently reheat to serve, being careful not to allow the soup to boil or the coconut milk will separate. Garnish with the freshly chopped cilantro.

* Asian foods stores generally carry fresh frozen lime leaves and Thai red curry paste.

— *Linda Gardner*

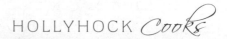

Caldeirada de Peixe —
Portuguese Fish Stew

The fish and shellfish can be varied in this dish, depending on your budget and what is available. The stew is best when made with fresh fish and homemade fish stock, but frozen fish and clam nectar will also work. Serve it with crusty bread or rolls and a crisp green salad. Try the Portuguese Rice Pudding (page 171) for dessert and you'll have an authentic Portuguese feast.

1. To prepare the seafood, cut the fish into 1½-inch cubes. Clean the mussels and/or clams. Shell the prawns or shrimp. Cut the cleaned squid into ½-inch rings. Refrigerate the prepared fish and shellfish.

2. In a large, heavy-bottomed pot, heat the olive oil, add the onions and sauté until softened. Add the bell peppers and sauté, stirring for a couple of minutes, until softened. Add the garlic and sauté briefly, stirring. Add the tomatoes, pimento paste, potatoes, paprika, bay leaf, fish stock and white wine. Bring to a boil, reduce heat and simmer until the potatoes are tender.

3. Add the fish and stir. Then add the shellfish, beginning with the clams and mussels, then the prawns/shrimp and finally the squid. Simmer gently, stirring, until the fish is opaque and the clams and mussels have opened their shells. Remove from heat and add the lemon juice, parsley and cilantro. Add salt and pepper to taste. Serve immediately.

VARIATIONS
You can use a variety of white, firm-fleshed fish such as cod, halibut, snapper, monkfish, sea bass and skate. Choose one or a mixture of two or three. Clams, mussels, prawns, shrimp and squid are delicious additions, but this stew is good with only fish as well.

* Portuguese pimento paste can be found in Portuguese and Mediterranean groceries. If you cannot find it, the stew will still be delicious. You can make a variation by combining canned roasted pimentos with a bit of salt and a touch of vinegar and some cayenne, in your blender or food processor.

— Hanyu Wasyliw

Serves 6-8

4 lbs.	fish and shellfish *	1.8 kg
½ cup	olive oil	120 mL
2 cups	medium diced onions	480 mL
1	diced green bell pepper	1
1	diced red bell pepper	1
1 tbsp	coarsely chopped garlic	15 mL
1½ cups	coarsely chopped tomatoes	360 mL
2 tbsp	hot Portuguese pimento paste *	30 mL
4-6 cups	peeled and cubed potatoes	1 - 1.5 L
3 tsp	paprika	15 mL
1	bay leaf	1
2 cups	fish/shellfish stock or clam nectar	480 mL
1½ cups	dry white wine	360 mL
¼ cup + 2 tbsp	fresh lemon juice	90 mL
½ cup	coarsely chopped parsley	120 mL
½ cup	coarsely chopped cilantro leaves	120 mL
	salt and pepper to taste	

Lemon-Lentil Soup

With classic Greek flavors, this soup is healthful and rich in protein. The lemon gives it a nice tang. Serve it with Savory Zucchini Muffins (page 144).

Serves 6-8

3 tbsp	sunflower or safflower oil	45 mL
2 cups	diced onions	480 mL
2 tbsp	crushed garlic	30 mL
1½ cups	finely diced carrots	360 mL
1 cup	diced potato, if desired	240 mL
2	bay leaves	2
1 cup	diced celery	240 mL
1 cup	dry red lentils	240 mL
5 cups	water or stock	1.2 L
⅓ cup	freshly squeezed lemon juice	80 mL
2 tbsp	chopped fresh dill	30 mL
4 cups	packed chopped fresh greens such as kale, chard, spinach, mustard, or sorrel	960 mL
	salt and pepper to taste	

1. In a soup pot, sauté the onions, garlic, carrots, potatoes and bay leaves in the oil just until the potatoes begin to soften, about 15 minutes.

2. Rinse and check the lentils for stones.

3. Add the celery and lentils to the soup pot and continue to sauté for 5 minutes. Add the water or stock and reduce the heat to medium. Cover and simmer until the lentils and all the vegetables are tender, approximately 15 minutes.

4. Just before serving, remove from the heat and stir in the lemon juice, chopped dill and greens. Stir until the greens have wilted. Season with salt and pepper to taste. Serve immediately.

— *Moreka Jolar*

"*The food at Hollyhock is always nourishing. It's so sane, like the atmosphere of the island.*"
— *Andrew Harvey*

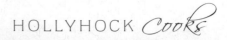

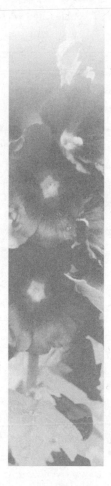

THREE

Entrées

IF EVERY DINNER IS A PERFORMANCE, and at Hollyhock every dinner truly is, then the entrée takes the leading role. It sets the tone for the side dishes, salads, special butters and desserts, which strive to bring out the best in the entrée, like a good supporting cast. Other dishes may quietly compete and sometimes steal the show, but generally it is the entrée that draws exclamations of anticipated pleasure from the lips of guests as they line up to serve themselves at the Hollyhock buffet. And generally, it is the entrée that brings people back to the table to fill their plates again.

The soil and the sea inspire Hollyhock's entrées. Vegetarian dishes, inspired by many cultures, contain varied ingredients and provide multiple textures, colors and flavors, as well as high nutritional value. Wild pink and sockeye salmon dressed in garden herbs and delicate flowers show up often on the Hollyhock buffet. Fresh halibut, oysters and prawns make guest performances. Culinarily charismatic and stunningly beautiful, Hollyhock's entrées are cooked from a philosophy that reveres beauty and puts pleasure first with fresh, local and organic food.

Baked Samosas

Samosa lovers, rejoice. Here is a way to cook those delicious pastry wraps without deep-frying them. Served with chutneys (page 98 and page 99) and Green Apple Raita (page 94), these samosas make eating Indian food at home the best treat in town.

Makes 16 small samosas

DOUGH

1⅓ cup	yogurt	320 mL
1 tbsp	grated fresh ginger	15 mL
½	seeded and finely minced jalapeño	½
1 tsp	salt	5 mL
2 cups	unbleached white flour	480 mL
1 cup	whole wheat flour	240 mL

FILLING

3 cups	diced potatoes	720 mL
2 cups	finely diced onions	480 mL
1½ cups	finely diced carrots	360 mL
¼ cup	freshly grated ginger	60 mL
2 tbsp	crushed garlic	30 mL
2 tbsp	whole coriander seeds, dry toasted and ground in a grinder	30 mL
1 tbsp	whole black mustard seeds	15 mL
	juice of ½ lemon	
	salt to taste	
1 cup	fresh or frozen peas	240 mL
¼ cup	melted butter	60 mL

1. In a medium-sized bowl, combine the yogurt with the ginger, jalapeño and salt. Add the white and whole wheat flour, stirring with a wooden spoon until the dough stiffens enough to work it with your hands. Knead the dough on a lightly floured surface until it becomes elastic, approximately 5 minutes. Cover with a damp towel and set it aside.

2. In a saucepan, cover the potatoes with plenty of water and boil them until they become tender. Drain and set aside. In a medium-sized frying pan, sauté the onions, carrots, ginger, garlic, whole mustard seeds and ground coriander until the carrot is tender. Add this mixture to the cooked potatoes. Stir in the lemon juice and salt to taste and fold in the peas.

3. Preheat the oven to 350°F. Divide the dough into 16 equal pieces. On a lightly floured surface, use a rolling pin to roll each piece of dough into a thin, round shape, approximately 5 inches in diameter. Place a scoop of filling on half of the circle of the dough. Fold the dough over to make a half-moon. Seal the edges well by pinching the dough together. Place the samosas on a lightly oiled cookie sheet. Brush the samosas with melted butter and bake at 350°F until they're brown, about 30-40 minutes. Serve warm. After shaping the samosas, you can also freeze them on a sheet and remove them from the freezer as desired. Bake immediately until golden and serve.

— *Rowan Brooks*

cook's tip

Use fresh ground spices whenever you can. We never know how long pre-ground spices have been on the shelf of a store and they loose their rich flavors over time. Purchase whole spices such as cardamom, cumin, black pepper, coriander etc. and grind them yourself in a spice or coffee grinder just before use. Taste the difference. And don't forget to always store your spices away from heat.

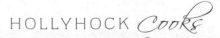

Barbecued Salmon with Mixed Garden Herbs

Fresh mayonnaise packed with fresh herbs is spread over the fish. The hot grill burns off the mayonnaise, infusing the salmon with moisture and the aroma of garden herbs. This dish is easy to prepare and very impressive.

1. Combine the mayonnaise, herbs, garlic and black pepper in a food processor until the herbs are finely ground. Spread evenly over flesh of the fillet and refrigerate for a minimum of 2 hours.

2. Preheat the barbecue. Lay the fillet, flesh down onto a well-oiled, hot grill and barbecue until the edges start to turn light pink and the fish has good dark stripes on it. Turn the fillet over carefully using 2 large spatulas and finish cooking with the skin-side down. Serve immediately.

VARIATION
The fillet can also be baked or a thin fillet can be broiled.

— *Moreka Jolar*

Serves 6-8

3 lbs.	single salmon fillet	1.4 kg
½ cup	Mayonnaise with Dijon and Tarragon (page 119) or commercial mayonnaise	120 mL
1 cup	mixed garden herbs, packed: basil, parsley, thyme, rosemary, marjoram, oregano, sage, tarragon	240 mL
1 tbsp	crushed garlic	15 mL
1 tsp	black pepper	5 mL

" *At the heart of Hollyhock's cuisine is the power of fresh food, the ocean, beach, garden and forest collaborating to provide us with living sustenance. Fresh, live food is what is meant to be, sustaining and directly infusing our bodies with the potent elements of our surroundings.* "
— *Gregor Robertson*

Barbecued Teriyaki Salmon

Marinating the salmon for a long time allows the classic sweet and salty tastes of a good teriyaki sauce to really penetrate the fish and will keep the salmon moist while barbecuing. Allow these salmon fillets to marinate for a minimum of 4 to 6 hours. All day or overnight is best. Serve this tender fish with fresh greens or Sautéed Hijiki Salad (page 20).

Serves 6-8

3 lbs.	salmon fillet	1.4 kg
2 tsp	crushed garlic	10 mL
2 tsp	freshly grated ginger	10 mL
1 cup	soy sauce	240 mL
1 cup	dry sherry	240 mL
¼ cup	sunflower or safflower oil	60 mL
1 tbsp	brown sugar	15 mL
	dash of chili oil or flakes	

1. Combine the garlic and ginger together and rub this mixture directly onto the flesh of the salmon fillet.

2. In a bowl, whisk together the soy sauce, sherry, oil, sugar and chili oil. Pour the marinade into the bottom of a baking dish that will neatly fit the fillet and lay the fish, flesh-down, into the marinade.

3. Preheat the barbecue. Barbecue the salmon on a very hot and pre-oiled grill. Start with flesh down on the grill until the edges start to cook and turn light pink. Carefully flip the fish with a large spatula and finish cooking with the skin down. As soon as the center or thickest portion of the fish flakes, it is done.

— *Jenica Rayne*

" *Food is the love gesture of the Earth and the Heavens.* "
— *Ann Mortifee*

 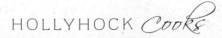

Purple Cabbage Slaw with Caraway and Currants page 23

Barbecued Salmon with Mixed
Garden Herbs page 49 and Mixed Vegetable
Marinade Salad with Raspberry Vinaigrette page 16

Top to bottom: Borscht page 35
Lemon-Lentil Soup page 46
Caldeirada de Peixe -
Portuguese Fish Stew page 45

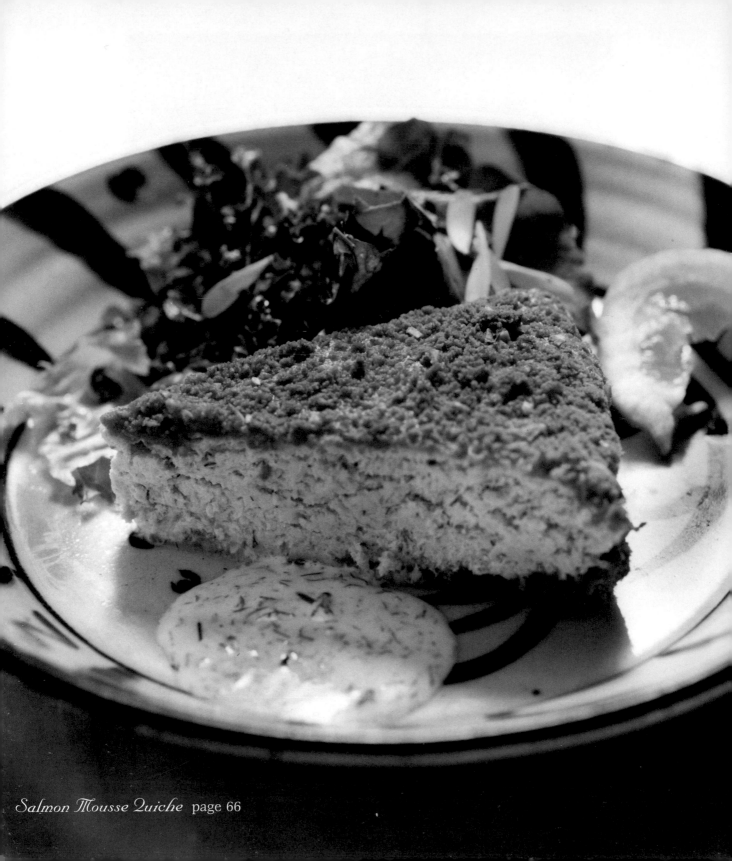

Salmon Mousse Quiche page 66

Clams or Mussels, Portuguese Style

In Portuguese, these are called "Ameijoas (clams) a Bulhao Pato," named after a 19th-century Portuguese poet, Senor Bulhao Pato. Nobody remembers his poetry but everyone in Portugal eats his clam dish. Perhaps he was a better chef than he was a poet. Serve with a crusty bread to sop up the juices, a young, fresh *vino verde* green wine from Portugal, and a crisp green salad from the garden for a simple and truly wonderful feast.

1. Scrub the shellfish clean and discard any shellfish that do not close with a bit of encouragement.

2. In a wok with a lid, or a large saucepan or frying pan, heat the olive oil over a medium-high heat. Add the garlic, jalapeños and salt. Stir for a minute or so until the garlic gives off its flavor. Throw the shellfish in and stir to coat with oil and garlic. Reduce heat to medium and cover the pot.

3. Allow it to cook for 1 to 2 minutes then stir the shellfish. Cook another 1 to 2 minutes and stir again. When most of the shells have opened, turn off the heat, stir to coat with oil and add the chopped herbs. Stir again, squeeze fresh lemon juice over it, stir and transfer into a serving dish with all the juices.

— *Hanyu Wasyliw*

Makes 4 appetizers or 2 main servings

2 lbs.	fresh live clams or mussels	915 g
¼ cup	olive oil	60 mL
4	peeled and roughly chopped garlic cloves	4
1	seeded and finely chopped jalapeño	1
½ tsp	coarse sea salt	2.5 mL
½ cup	chopped cilantro or Italian parsley	120 mL
½	lemon	½

Caponata with Serpentini Pasta

Caponata is a traditional Italian relish and is often served as a starter or antipasto with crackers. Here is it served as a thick and richly flavored sauce over the twisty serpentini pasta. Serpentini pasta is named after the serpent because of its snake-like shape. Other pasta will also work well in this recipe.

8-10 servings

1 lb.	serpentini pasta	460 g
4 cups	cubed eggplant	960 mL
2 cups	diced onion	480 mL
1 tbsp	minced garlic	15 mL
1 cup	coarsely chopped celery	240 mL
1 cup	cubed young yellow zucchini	240 mL
2 cups	assorted bell peppers, cut in large chunks	480 mL
3 cups	cubed fresh tomatoes	720 mL
¼ cup	red wine, if desired	60 mL
¼ cup	rinsed capers	60 mL
½ tsp	black pepper	2.5 mL
½ tsp	red chili flakes	2.5 mL
2	bay leaves	2
1 cup	spicy green olives, cut in rounds	240 mL
½ cup	pitted and coarsely chopped black olives, such as Moroccan or Kalamata	120 mL

1. In a deep saucepan, sauté the eggplant, onion, garlic and celery in olive oil for about 10 minutes or until the celery starts to get tender. Add the zucchini, peppers, tomato, red wine, capers, black pepper, chili flakes and bay leaves. Cover and allow it to simmer for 45-50 minutes, until it forms a thick, cooked sauce.

2. While the caponata is simmering, cook the pasta according to the instructions.

3. Add the green and black olives to the sauce.

4. Top each serving of pasta with a generous scoop of caponata. Try adding a handful of lightly toasted pine nuts to the caponata and top with grated cheese.

— *Moreka Jolar*

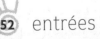

Cauliflower and Quinoa Bake

Quinoa was one of the ancient staple foods of the Incas and was known as the Mother Grain. Compared with other grains, quinoa is higher in protein, is an excellent source of iron, and contains more calcium than milk. Serve this delicious dish with Yellow Beans with Honey Balsamic Vinaigrette and Oven-Roasted Cherry Tomatoes (page 25) for a colorful meal.

Preheat the oven to 350°F.

1. In a large saucepan, begin by sautéeing the onions, leeks and garlic in the oil until the onion is transparent, approximately 10 minutes. Add the cauliflower, stir and cover, allowing the cauliflower to steam for 5 minutes.

2. Remove from the heat and transfer it to a very large bowl. Add all the remaining ingredients and stir well.

3. Gently press into a lightly oiled 9x13-inch baking dish. Sprinkle a bit of paprika over the top. Bake at 350°F for 30-40 minutes. Serve hot.

— *Moreka Jolar*

8-10 servings

2 tbsp	sunflower or safflower oil	30 mL
3 cups	diced onion	720 mL
3	chopped and rinsed leeks	3
1 tbsp	crushed garlic	15 mL
1	coarsely chopped cauliflower head	1
	juice of 1 lemon	
1 tsp	chopped fresh dill	5 mL
1 cup	pitted and coarsely chopped Kalamata olives	240 mL
¼ cup	chopped fresh parsley	60 mL
1 tsp	black pepper	5 mL
½ tsp	salt	2.5 mL
2 cups	grated sharp cheddar, Swiss, Gouda or crumbled feta	480 mL
2 cups	cooked quinoa, or rice, bulgur or millet	480 mL
	paprika to garnish	

 cook's tip

Quinoa is easy to prepare. Rinse 1 cup of dry quinoa, then place the quinoa and 2 cups of water in a small saucepan. Cover and bring it to a boil, then reduce to simmer until the quinoa absorbs the water, approximately 15-20 minutes. Remove the lid and fluff with a fork.

Chèvre Tart

For the sophisticated taste of a Parisian café, serve this creamy and extravagantly
rich tart with a salad dressed with Hollyhock Poppyseed Dressing (page 31)
or Green Goddess Dressing (page 28) and a freshly baked baguette.

8-10 servings

CRUST

	soft butter	
½ cup	fine breadcrumbs	120 mL
½ cup	finely ground walnuts or hazelnuts	120 mL

FILLING

8 oz.	soft chèvre	230 g
4 oz.	soft cream cheese	115 g
2 tsp	chopped garlic	10 mL
3	eggs	3
½ tsp	salt	2.5 mL
1 tsp	freshly ground black pepper	5 mL
1 tbsp	finely chopped fresh tarragon	15 mL
1 tbsp	chopped fresh basil	15 mL
2 tbsp	chopped fresh chives	30 mL

Preheat the oven to 350°F.

1. Generously grease an 8-inch springform pan, being sure to cover the bottom and sides with soft butter. To prepare the crust, mix the breadcrumbs and chopped nuts together in a small bowl and then sprinkle on to the bottom and sides of the pan. Pat down and refrigerate.

2. To prepare the filling, place the chèvre, cream cheese, garlic, eggs and salt in a food processor. Blend briefly, using the pulse button and scraping the sides of the bowl, until the ingredients are well mixed. Add the pepper and herbs and blend briefly.

3. Remove the crust from the refrigerator and pour in the cheese mixture. Bake until set, about 30-40 minutes. Allow it to cool on a cooling rack. Serve at room temperature or cold.

— Carmen Rosse

Halibut with Lime-Miso Marinade

This succulent marinade infuses halibut with bold and exotic flavors. It's best when marinated overnight so it can soak well through the thick fillet. Roasted Barley Pilaf with Mushrooms and Hazelnuts (page 91) makes an excellent dinner companion to this recipe.

1. Blend all the marinade ingredients well and then spread the mixture evenly over the flesh of the halibut. The fish can remain in 1 piece or be portioned. Cover and marinate for at least 6 hours or preferably overnight in the refrigerator. Use a rubber spatula to scrape most of the marinade off the fish and reserve it.

2. In a very hot frying pan with the oil, sear the top (not the skin side) of the fish until it is well browned. Turn the fish over in the pan, reduce the heat to medium and add the remaining marinade, cover and cook just until the halibut flakes at the center and is white through. Serve immediately, garnished with thinly sliced scallions.

* Mirin is sweetened rice vinegar and Sake is Japanese rice wine.

— *Moreka Jolar*

Serves 6

3 lbs.	halibut fillet	1.4 kg
3 tbsp	sunflower or safflower oil	45 mL

MARINADE

⅓ cup	miso paste	80 mL
⅓ cup	mirin or Sake *	80 mL
¼ cup	freshly grated ginger	60 mL
	zest and juice from 1 lime	
1	scallion	1

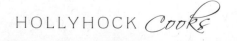

Cod Dijonnaise

Offer this baked fish on a bed of fresh kale leaves with Middle Eastern Flatbread (page 135) or pita (page 140) to soak up the wonderful sauce. For vegetarians, this recipe is also delicious with firm tofu instead of fish.

Serves 6

3 lbs.	cod fillet, or other firm-fleshed white fish, such as red snapper or halibut	1.4 kg
¼ cup	melted butter	60 mL
½ cup	liquid honey	120 mL
¼ cup	prepared Dijon mustard or hot mustard powder	60 mL
I tsp	curry powder, or 2 tsp Fresh Curry Paste (pg 107)	5 mL

Preheat the oven to 350°F.

1. Cut the fish into 6 serving-sized portions. Sauté the fish pieces briefly in the melted butter in a medium-hot pan, searing both sides of the fish.

2. Combine the honey, mustard and curry powder in a small bowl with a whisk.

3. Arrange the fish pieces in the bottom of a baking dish and then pour the sauce over them. Bake at 350°F for 10-20 minutes, depending on the thickness of the fish, or until the fish flakes at the center but is not dry.

VARIATION

Use firm tofu instead of the fish and follow the same steps.

— *Debra Fontaine*

Tomato Crowned Cod

Basil and tomato come together to crown the cod with the inseparable goodness of fruit and herb. Crunchy seasoned breadcrumbs top off sweet baked tomatoes and peppers, all of which rest on a perfect tender fillet of cod. The cod can be baked as one fillet or portioned into 6 to 8 fillets before baking. Serve with a side dish of Roasted Roots with Lemon and Rosemary (page 92).

6-8 servings

3 lbs.	cod fillet	1.4 kg
I	lemon	I
2 cups	Roma tomatoes, sliced in thin rounds	480 mL
⅓ cup	minced yellow bell pepper	80 mL
⅓ cup	minced onion	80 mL
¼ tsp	salt	1.2 mL
¼ tsp	pepper	1.2 mL
½ cup	breadcrumbs	120 mL
2 tbsp	olive oil	30 mL
2 tbsp	chopped fresh basil	30 mL

Preheat the oven to 400°F.

1. Lay the cod fillet on a lightly oiled baking dish and squeeze the lemon juice onto the fillet. Arrange the tomato rounds on top of the fish.

2. In a small bowl, mix the bell pepper, onion, salt and pepper, and sprinkle over the tomato.

3. Use that same small bowl to combine the breadcrumbs with the olive oil and basil and sprinkle on the very top. Bake for 15-20 minutes, depending on the thickness of the fish. The fish is done when it flakes at the center.

— *Rosemary Wooldridge*

Curried Summer Squash
Half-Moon Bouquet

This is a visually beautiful meal. Beets change the color of the flesh of the squash, but not the skin, which naturally highlights each half-moon with a band of iridescent yellow. The nuts give a great contrasting texture, and the goat cheese irresistibly melds everything together for a deliciously magical meal. Serve this spicy and creamy dish on a bed of Fragrant Saffron Rice (page 85), with Mango Chutney (page 99) and a salad.

Serves 4

3	medium beets peeled	3
¾ cup	water	180 mL
2 tbsp	olive oil	30 mL
1 cup	chopped onions	240 mL
3	small to medium yellow summer squash such as zucchini or pattypan	3
½ cup	slivered or finely sliced toasted almonds	120 mL
½ tsp	sesame oil	2.5 mL
¼ cup	sesame seeds	60 mL
1	small dried and finely diced red chili pepper	1
1½ tsp	Madras curry powder	7.5 mL
¼ cup	crumbled soft garlic herbed chèvre	60 mL
3 cups	chopped fresh beet greens, packed	720 mL
	sea salt to taste	

1. Cut the beets into thin strips and cook them in a medium-sized saucepan with ½ cup of water, covered tightly. Cook until tender. Drain and set aside.

2. In a wok or large skillet, sauté the onions in the olive oil on medium heat until just before they become transparent.

3. While the onions are cooking, slice the squash lengthwise and then slice it into ¼-inch-thick half moons. Add the squash to the onions and cook until the squash just begins to get tender but not mushy. Add the almonds, sesame oil, sesame seeds, chili pepper and curry powder. Toss lightly to mix and continue to sauté a moment. Blend the chèvre gently into the mixture. Add ¼ cup of water and the beet greens and cover and allow them to steam lightly. When the greens are barely limp add the beets to the mixture and season with salt to taste. You can add more water now if you'd like a more soupy consistency.

— *Carol Newell*

Filo Bake with Leeks and Shiitake Mushrooms

Luxurious, extravagant and rich are perfect words to describe this filo pastry pie with its fusion of tastes. Portions can be small. Serve it with a fresh green salad.

Serves 10-12

¾ cup	olive oil	180 mL
5 cups	dry shiitake mushrooms	1.2 L
6 cups	sliced white mushrooms (approx. 1 lb.)	1.4 L
6 cups	thinly sliced and rinsed leeks	1.4 L
1½ tbsp	minced garlic	23 mL
1 tbsp	black pepper	15 mL
1 tsp	salt	5 mL
2 tbsp	fresh thyme	30 mL
¼ cup	dry white wine	60 mL
2 cups	ricotta or cottage cheese	480 mL
1 cup	grated Parmesan	240 mL
3	eggs	3
½ cup	chopped fresh parsley	120 mL
1 cup	grated smoked Gruyère	240 mL
12 sheets	filo pasty	12 sheets
½ cup	melted butter	120 mL

Preheat the oven to 350°F.

1. Cover the dry shiitake mushrooms with boiling water and soak them for at least 1 hour. Drain off the water and thinly slice them.

2. In a medium-sized frying pan, sauté the shitake mushrooms in 4 tbsp of olive oil until golden. Set aside in a large bowl.

3. Use the same frying pan to sauté the white mushrooms in 4 tbsp olive oil until they reduce in size and turn golden, approximately 15 minutes. Add them to the shiitake mushrooms.

4. In the same frying pan, gently sauté the leeks in 4 tbsp of olive oil with the garlic, salt, pepper, fresh thyme and wine. Add the leek mixture to the mushrooms and toss it all together well.

5. In a small bowl, whisk together the ricotta or cottage cheese, Parmesan, eggs and parsley. Add this to the leek and mushroom mixture and combine well.

6. Use a pastry brush to brush a 9x12-inch deep baking dish with melted butter and layer 6 sheets of filo, brushing melted butter over each sheet as you layer it. Pour the filling onto the pastry and spread evenly into the bottom of the pan. Top the filling with the grated Gruyère. Layer the remaining 6 sheets of filo pastry on top of this, repeating the method of brushing each sheet with melted butter. Use a sharp knife to score the top pastry layers into 10-12 equal portions. This prevents the fragile pastry from crumbling after baking. Bake for 30-45 minutes or until the top of the pastry is very golden and flaky. Allow it to sit for 10-15 minutes before serving.

— *Moreka Jolar*

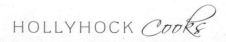

Herbed Polenta Torta with Spinach and Mushrooms

Polenta is a mainstay in parts of Italy. It is simply the result of cooking cornmeal and water into a kind of hot cereal. Here is it baked and served as a base for this rustic, hearty and fulfilling tort. Omit the cheeses and substitute grated or crumbled firm tofu for a nondairy delicacy.

1. To make the polenta, combine the yellow cornmeal, bell pepper, parsley, oregano, basil, salt and black pepper in a large saucepan. Whisk the ingredients while adding the water. Place the pot over medium heat, continue to whisk while bringing the polenta to a boil and then reduce the heat and simmer for 15 minutes. Remove the saucepan from the heat and stir in the Parmesan cheese. Pour into a 10-inch greased springform pan, spreading it evenly. Cool until completely firm, approximately 2 hours at room temperature.

2. Preheat the oven to 350°F.

3. For the topping, sauté the mushrooms, zucchini, yellow squash, onions, garlic, red wine and tomatoes in a large skillet until the vegetables are tender and most of the liquid has evaporated. Transfer to a bowl. Add the artichoke hearts, spinach and ricotta, or tofu, and beaten eggs. Spread this topping over the polenta, arrange the tomato rounds over the top, and cover with the mozzarella cheese. Bake at 350°F for approximately 1 hour or until the top has set. It should be firm when you shake it gently. Allow it to cool on a rack for 15 minutes before serving.

— *Moreka Jolar*

8-10 servings

POLENTA

1¼ cup	yellow cornmeal	300 mL
½ cup	diced red bell pepper	120 mL
¼ cup	chopped fresh parsley	60 mL
1 tsp	chopped fresh oregano	5 mL
1 tsp	chopped fresh basil	5 mL
¾ tsp	salt	4 mL
¼ tsp	black pepper	1.5 mL
4 cups	water	960 mL
¼ cup	freshly grated Parmesan	60 mL

TOPPING

2 cups	sliced mushrooms	480 mL
1 cup	thinly sliced zucchini	240 mL
1 cup	thinly sliced yellow summer squash such as pattypan	240 mL
1 cup	diced onions	240 mL
2 tbsp	crushed garlic	30 mL
¼ cup	dry red wine	60 mL
1 cup	chopped fresh tomatoes	240 mL
1 cup	chopped artichoke hearts	240 mL
2 cups	blanched, drained and chopped spinach	480 mL
1 cup	ricotta cheese or crumbled tofu	240 mL
3	eggs, beaten	3
1 cup	shredded mozzarella	240 mL
2 cups	thickly sliced tomato rounds	480 mL

Mediterranean Garlic Custard Tart

The process of poaching the garlic in milk in this recipe reveals all the natural sugar hidden away in the garlic. This gives the tart a pleasant and aromatic sweet edge. This savory, cheesy pie is very creamy and elegant.

Serves 8-10

I batch	Single Crust Basic Whole Wheat Pastry (see page 123)	
2	heads of garlic, cloves peeled and lightly smashed	2
1½ cup	milk	360 mL
I	medium eggplant	I
3	eggs beaten	3
4-6	sliced scallions	4-6
I	roasted and diced red bell pepper *	I
I	small bunch of fresh basil and/or parsley	I
I cup	freshly grated Romano, Gruyère or Parmesan cheese	240 mL
¼ tsp	salt	1.2 mL
¼ tsp	black pepper	1.2 mL
½ cup	sliced and pitted Kalamata olives, if desired	120 mL

1. Place the garlic cloves and milk in a small pot. Bring to a simmer, being careful not to boil. Poach the garlic on a very low heat for approximately 20 minutes. Remove from the heat and allow the mixture to cool to lukewarm.

2. Score the skin of the eggplant by running the sharp prongs of a fork into and along the entire surface of the eggplant. This helps the tough skin to soften while cooking. Cut it in ½-inch-thick rounds. Sauté the eggplant rounds with a little olive oil in a large skillet until lightly browned on both sides and very soft.

3. Remove the garlic from the milk with a slotted spoon, and mash with a potato masher. Whisk together the milk and garlic with the beaten eggs.

4. In a small skillet, sauté the scallions in butter or oil until softened. Add this to the milk mixture. Mix in the diced red bell pepper to this mixture.

5. Chop or tear the basil leaves and chop the parsley. Add it to the milk mixture. Mix in ½ cup of the grated cheese. Add salt and pepper.

6. Preheat the oven to 350°F. Make the pastry according to the instructions and roll it out with a rolling pin on a lightly floured surface. Place it in a 9-inch pie plate or quiche dish and cut the edges to fit. Lay the eggplant slices on the pastry shell. Sprinkle Kalamata olive pieces, if desired. Pour the custard mixture over it and sprinkle the top with the remaining ½ cup of cheese. Bake until the custard is set, approximately 30 to 40 minutes. A knife should come out of the center clean. This is best served warm or at room temperature.

* Roasted bell peppers are widely available in large groceries and delis or see page 104 for instructions on roasting your own.

— *Elena Fraser*

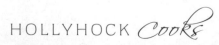

Mussels in White Wine and Dijon Cream

Mussels make a romantic dish for a picnic on the beach under the stars, or even at the kitchen table. These mussels are steamed in wine, which is then reduced with cream and smooth Dijon mustard for an elegant and fine feast. Serve this dish with a crusty bread to soak up the juices, and a crisp green salad.

1. Rinse the mussels well and scrub the shells clean with a brush. Put the wine and mussels in a large saucepan. Cover and steam until the shellfish open. Remove the mussels with a slotted spoon and keep them covered in a bowl.

2. Add the cream and mustard to the wine and continue to cook on low heat for approximately 20 minutes, or until the mixture begins to thicken. Add the fresh thyme. Pour the cream, wine and mustard mixture over the mussels. Serve immediately.

— *Debra Fontaine*

Serves 4-5

4 lbs.	fresh live mussels	1.8 kg
2 cups	dry white wine	480 mL
1 cup	heavy cream	240 mL
1 tsp	prepared Dijon mustard	5 mL
	pinch of fresh thyme	

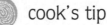 cook's tip

Discard any open shellfish that won't close with a bit of encouragement. These are not fresh and are no longer safe to eat.

Mussels with Chipotle Sauce

These spicy mussels will make your dinner sizzle. The chipotle sauce gives a fragrant and smoky flavor to the shellfish. You can cook this dish with clams instead of mussels, depending on what's available. Serve with a green salad and Roasted Garlic Focaccia (page 141) to soak up all of the juices.

Serves 4-5

4 lbs.	fresh live mussels	1.8 kg
¼ cup	tamari	60 mL
1 tbsp	crushed garlic	15 mL
	zest and juice of 2 limes	
1	whole chipotle pepper in adobo sauce *	1
½ cup	packed chopped fresh cilantro	120 mL

1. Rinse and scrub the mussel shells. Discard any open mussels that won't close when you press their shells together, as these are no longer good to eat.

2. Combine the tamari, garlic, lime zest, lime juice and chipotle in a blender until well blended. Heat this sauce in a deep saucepan until simmering. Add the mussels and toss until covered with the sauce.

3. Cover and cook on medium-high heat until every shell is open. Toss together a few more times. Transfer to a serving bowl, sprinkle with fresh cilantro and serve immediately.

* Chipotle peppers are smoked jalapeños and available in small tins of adobo sauce in most Mexican foods sections.

— *Moreka Jolar*

Nut Loaf

Nut loaf is tastier than meatloaf and more nutritious. Serve this hearty, protein-packed entrée with Miso or Nut Butter Gravy (page 100) and Sesame Home Fries (page 94). The egg can be omitted for a vegan loaf.

Preheat the oven to 350°F.

1. In a large frying pan, sauté the onion, celery, mushrooms and all the fresh herbs and spices in the oil until tender. Transfer the mixture to a large bowl and combine with cooked rice, chopped nuts, crumbled tofu and egg. Mix well.

2. Lightly oil all the sides of a loaf pan and layer the bottom with slivered almonds. Press the loaf ingredients into the pan and bake at 350°F for approximately 1 hour. Allow the loaf to cool for 15 minutes before running a knife around all the edges to loosen it from the pan. Invert onto a serving plate. Serve immediately.

— *Moreka Jolar*

Serves 8-10

2 tbsp	sunflower or safflower oil	30 mL
1 cup	diced onion	240 mL
1 cup	diced celery	240 mL
1 cup	sliced mushrooms	240 mL
¼ cup	chopped fresh parsley	60 mL
1 tbsp	chopped fresh basil	15 mL
1 tbsp	chopped fresh marjoram	15 mL
1 tbsp	Spike or other vegetable salt	15 mL
1 tsp	chopped fresh rosemary	5 mL
1 tsp	black pepper	5 mL
2 cups	cooked brown rice	480 mL
12 oz.	soft crumbled tofu	340 g
2 cups	toasted and finely chopped almonds	480 mL
1	egg	1
¼ cup	slivered almonds	60 mL

 cook's tip

Always use fresh herbs. If these aren't available to you, a half portion of the dry herb will do. For example, 1 tbsp of chopped fresh basil equals ½ tbsp dry.

 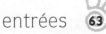

Prawns with Roasted
Red Pepper Sauce

Here are two easy ways to please the prawn-lover. The first method, using a wok, is fast, easy, delicious and fresh. The second way, with the broiler, gives the prawns a roasted flavor. Both use a sweet and smoky sauce that has a spicy edge.

Serves 6-8

3 lbs.	fresh prawn tails, shelled or not	1.4 kg
2 tbsp	sunflower or safflower oil	30 mL
1 batch	Roasted Red Pepper Sauce (page 104)	1 batch
1 bunch	chopped cilantro, parsley or scallions, for garnish	1 bunch

IN A WOK

1. Heat the oil in a large wok. Add the Roasted Red Pepper Sauce and cook on medium-high heat until bubbly, stirring with a wooden spoon. Add the prawns, toss to cover with the sauce, and continue to cook on high heat, stirring often. Cook until the prawns curl and the shells turn pink. Prawns cook very fast, taking approximately 3 minutes, and shelled prawns will cook even faster. Taste 1 to test them for readiness. Serve immediately, garnished with fresh herbs or scallions.

IN A BROILER

1. In a small bowl, cover the prawns completely with the Roasted Red Pepper Sauce and then spread them out in a lightly oiled cake or casserole pan. Place them under the broiler and cook until the shells begin to roast. Toss them to roast the other sides, being careful not to overcook. them Remove and garnish with fresh herbs or scallions. Serve immediately.

— *Moreka Jolar*

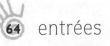

Roasted Vegetable Lasagne

Hearty and sweet, this lasagne has less tomato sauce than is traditionally used and is filled with vegetables. The roasted vegetables make this lasagne unique and elegant.

Preheat the oven to 400°F.

1. Cut the peppers in half length-wise. Seed them and lay them out on a cookie sheet with the skin side up. Roast them at 400°F or broil them until their skins have blackened. Place the peppers in a bowl and cover it with plastic wrap and allow them to cool.

2. Reduce oven to 375°F. Slice each zucchini lengthwise into 3 or 4 wide strips. Score the eggplant's skin by running the sharp tongs of a fork into and along the skin of the entire fruit and slice lengthwise into ¼-inch-thick slices. Lay the zucchini and eggplant on a lightly oiled baking sheet, brush each piece with oil and roast at 375°F until tender and brown.

3. Reduce the oven to 350°F. Peel the bell peppers and set aside. In a small bowl, whisk together the ricotta, eggs, oregano and black pepper.

4. To assemble, spread a thin layer of tomato sauce in the bottom of a lightly oiled 9x12-inch deep baking dish. Follow with:
   - A layer of uncooked lasagne noodles
   - Half the cheese mixture, evenly spread over the noodles
   - Roasted eggplant, whole flanks arranged over the cheese
   - Another layer of noodles
   - 3 to 4 cups of the tomato sauce, spread over noodles
   - Roasted zucchini, whole strips arranged over tomato sauce
   - Remaining half of cheese mix, spread evenly over the zucchini
   - A final layer of noodles
   - Whole roasted bell peppers, spread out over the noodles
   - Remaining tomato sauce, spread over the peppers
   - Top with the grated mozzarella.

5. Bake the lasagne uncovered for about 1½ hours. The cheese on top will be golden and bubbly. If you do not want the cheese to brown, cover the top of the lasagne with aluminum foil during the last half-hour of baking. Allow it to cool and set for 20 minutes before serving.

— *Moreka Jolar*

Serves 12-16

1 lb.	uncooked lasagne noodles	460 g
5	red or yellow bell peppers	5
3	large zucchinis	3
1	eggplant	1
¼ cup	olive oil	60 mL
3 cups	ricotta or low-fat cottage cheese	720 mL
2	eggs beaten	2
2 tsp	chopped fresh oregano	10 mL
1 tsp	black pepper	5 mL
7 cups	Sweet Basil Tomato Sauce (see page 105)	1.7 L
2 cups	grated mozzarella	480 mL

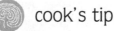

cook's tip

For a non-dairy lasagne, omit the mozzarella and crumble medium-firm tofu in place of the ricotta. Cooked wheat-free pasta will also work very well in this recipe.

Salmon Polenta Casserole

Here is an easy and fast way to use up leftover fish. Pleasing to all ages, this is a good, nutritious, homestyle casserole.

Serves 6-8

2 cups	milk	480 mL
2 tbsp	butter	30 mL
1 tsp	salt	5 mL
¾ cup	yellow cornmeal	180 mL
1 cup	cooked flaked salmon	240 mL
¼ cup	minced onion	60 mL
¼ cup	diced red bell pepper	60 mL
¼ cup	diced green bell pepper	60 mL
4	eggs separated	4
	fresh parsley to garnish	

Preheat the oven to 375°F.

1. In a medium-sized saucepan, bring the milk, butter and salt to a gentle boil. Lower the heat and slowly add the cornmeal, stirring constantly until thickened, approximately 1 minute. Remove from the heat. Add the flaked salmon, onion, bell peppers and egg yolks. Whisk together well.

2. In a medium-sized bowl, whip the egg whites with an electric mixer until they are stiff. Fold the egg whites well into the polenta mixture. Turn the polenta mixture into a lightly oiled 8x9-inch casserole dish. Bake at 375°F for approximately 30 minutes. Garnish with fresh parsley. Serve hot with a green salad.

— *Debra Fontaine*

Salmon Mousse Quiche

Silky salmon mousse meets warm quiche for a mouth-wateringly delicious dish. Both the tart shell and the quiche are simple to prepare, with elegant results and a mild taste.

Serves 8-10

1	Savory Nut Tart Shell (page 143)	1

FILLING

2 cups	cooked flaked salmon	480 mL
1 cup	yogurt	240 mL
3	eggs	3
¼ cup	diced onion	60 mL
1 tsp	chopped fresh dill	5 mL
	a dash of hot sauce such as Tabasco	

Preheat the oven to 350°F.

1. Reserve 1 cup of the Savory Nut Tart Shell mixture and press the rest into the bottom of a lightly oiled 9-inch pie plate.

2. Combine all the filling ingredients in a food processor until blended, approximately 10 seconds. Pour this over the uncooked tart shell. Sprinkle the remaining tart shell ingredients over the top. This will be a light covering. Bake the quiche until the center is firm when you shake it gently, approximately 45 minutes. Cool for 15 minutes before cutting to serve.

— *Debra Fontaine*

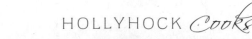

Savory Yam Cakes

Great as an appetizer for an Indian meal, these sweet yet savory cakes make a light and fanciful dish. They can be served as a light and elegant starter or combined with Green Beans Indian Style (page 88) to make a light meal. Serve them with Mango Chutney (page 99) or raita (page 94).

1. Toast the cumin seeds in a small frying pan just until brown.

2. In a medium-sized bowl whip the eggs before mixing in all the remaining ingredients, including the toasted cumin seeds. Combine well. Use a spoon to drop the batter into a large, hot, lightly oiled frying pan and cook slowly on each side until each cake is very golden, about 25 minutes. Keep these warm under a tea towel while cooking the remaining cakes.

— *Moreka Jolar*

Makes 12 small cakes

½ tsp	whole cumin seeds	2.5 mL
4	eggs	4
5 cups	grated yam	1.2 L
1 cup	grated onion	240 mL
¾ cup	chopped fresh cilantro	180 mL
3 tsp	freshly diced red chili or 1 tsp ground	15 mL
1 tsp	salt	5 mL
1 tsp	pepper	5 mL

"When food is prepared with the kind of care that we lavish on a beloved child, it feeds our good hearts and nourishes not only our own lives, but also what we can contribute to the world."
— *Joan Borysenko*

Shrimp and Braised Leek Tart

This rich and rustic tart is best served next to a mixed green salad dressed
in Green Goddess Dressing (page 28). The salty Romano cheese
complements the shrimp perfectly.

Serves 8

I batch	Single Crust Basic Whole Wheat Pastry (page 123)	I batch
2 tbsp	olive oil	30 mL
3	large leeks finely chopped and rinsed	3
2 tsp	crushed garlic	10 mL
I cup	chopped red bell pepper	240 mL
I tsp	fresh thyme	5 mL
I tsp	black pepper	5 mL
I tbsp	chopped fresh parsley	15 mL
3	eggs	3
I cup	yogurt	240 mL
½ tsp	salt	2.5 mL
½ cup	grated Romano cheese	120 mL
I cup	cooked shrimp	240 mL

1. In a medium-sized frying pan, slowly braise the leeks in the olive oil until they are beginning to brown. Add the garlic, bell pepper, thyme, black pepper and parsley. Cook just until the bell pepper is tender and set aside.

2. Preheat the oven to 350°F. On a lightly floured surface, use a rolling pin to roll out the pastry, lay it into a 9-inch pie plate or quiche dish and cut to fit.

3. In a small bowl, whip the eggs, yogurt and salt with a whisk until foamy. Spread the grated Romano cheese evenly over the uncooked pastry in the pie plate. Cover with the leek mixture and then the shrimp. Pour the egg mixture over this and bake until firm when shaken, about 30-45 minutes. Allow it to cool for 15 minutes before slicing. Garnish with sprigs of thyme.

— Moreka Jolar

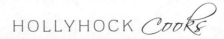

Soba Noodles with Ginger-Miso Eggplant

These Japanese hearty buckwheat noodles make a fine match for meaty eggplant. Tangy and spicy, they're sensational topped with toasted and ground sesame seeds.

1 In a large saucepan, add the soba noodles to a generous portion of boiling water and cook them until tender. Drain and set aside.

2. Using a medium-sized wok, sauté the eggplant and onions in the oil on high heat, stirring often. Cook until the eggplant is soft and tender, approximately 15 minutes. Add the bell pepper and Ginger-Miso Sauce and continue to cook for another 5 minutes. Remove from heat.

3. Add the cooked soba noodles to the wok, toss well and serve garnished with scallions and a lemon wedge.

— *Moreka Jolar*

Serves 6-8

10 oz.	soba noodles	285 g
1 batch	Ginger-Miso Sauce (pg 102)	1 batch
2 tbsp	sunflower or safflower oil	30 mL
4 cups	cubed eggplant	960 mL
2 cups	thinly sliced onions	480 mL
1 cup	chopped red bell pepper	240 mL
4	chopped scallions to garnish	4
1	lemon cut in wedges	1

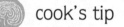 cook's tip

Any time you're cooking eggplant either peel or run a fork along the length of the eggplant, piercing the skin before cooking it. This enables the tough skin of the eggplant to tenderize while cooking.

Cold Tangy Orchid Noodles

These traditional Asian flavors infuse the Chinese noodles over time. The noodles will keep refrigerated for four to five days and are best served after having had an entire day to marinate. Make this cold noodle dish your own by adding your favorite thinly sliced and brightly colored vegetables, such as red and yellow peppers, snow peas or peanuts.

Serves 8-10

1 lb.	fresh, fat Chinese egg noodles *	460 g
3½ tbsp	sesame oil	53 mL
3½ tbsp	dark soy sauce	53 mL
2 tbsp	sugar	30 mL
1½ tbsp	balsamic vinegar	23 mL
2 tsp	coarse salt	10 mL
	hot chili oil to taste	
½ cup	thinly sliced scallions	120 mL

1. Cook the noodles according to the package directions. Drain and set them aside.

2. Mix the seasonings together with a whisk in a small bowl. Toss the seasonings with the noodles. Add the scallions. Place the noodles in a large bowl, cover it with plastic wrap and let it marinate at room temperature for at least 3 hours. Refrigerate.

* These noodles are sometimes known as Shanghai noodles and are found fresh or frozen in Asian food sections.

— *Debra Fontaine*

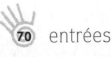

Spaghetti with Black Olive Pistou

Traditional French pistou is similar to Italian pesto and is a paste of basil, garlic and olive oil. This recipe has the same principle, but highlights black olives and anchovies for an intensely flavored twist on an old standard.

1. Process the olives, olive oil, garlic and anchovy paste in a food processor to make a finely ground paste. Set aside.

2. Cook the spaghetti according to instructions and drain. Toss the pistou paste with the hot spaghetti and serve immediately.

— *Chloe Gregg*

Serves 4-6

1 lb.	spaghetti	460 g
4 cups	sliced California black olives	960 mL
½ cup	olive oil	120 mL
2 tbsp	crushed garlic	30 mL
1 tbsp	anchovy paste	15 mL

Mediterranean Pasta

With basil, black olives, feta cheese and more, this pasta is bold and intensely flavored. The tang of wine vinegar and the feta complement the sweet tomatoes perfectly.

1. In a large bowl, combine the tomatoes, olives, basil, olive oil, vinegar, garlic and chili flakes.

2. Cook the pasta according to the instructions.

3. Add the hot cooked pasta to the bowl containing the sauce. Toss well and top with the feta cheese. Serve.

— *Chloe Gregg*

8-10 servings

1 lb.	linguini or angel hair pasta	460 g
4 cups	fresh cubed red or sweet yellow tomatoes	960 mL
1 cup	sliced California black olives	240 mL
¼ cup	chopped fresh basil	60 mL
3 tbsp	olive oil	45 mL
3 tbsp	red wine vinegar	45 mL
1 tbsp	crushed garlic	15 mL
½ tsp	red chili flakes	2.5 mL
1 cup	crumbled feta cheese	240 mL

Spanakopita with Green Olives and Artichoke Hearts

Spanakopita is traditional Greek spinach pie made with feta cheese and filo pastry. This variation on a Greek favorite presents a wonderful opportunity to use greens of every kind to form delightful crisp triangles. Working with filo pastry can be a delicate matter, but don't be intimidated. You'll get better as you handle the pastry and it will be well worth the effort.

Serves 10

10 cups	packed spinach or fresh chard	2.4 L
2 cups	finely diced onions	480 mL
2 tbsp	minced garlic	30 mL
2 tbsp	chopped fresh oregano	30 mL
I tsp	pepper	5 mL
2 cups	coarsely chopped artichoke hearts	480 mL
2 cups	crumbled feta	480 mL
I cup	sliced green olives	240 mL
I tsp	chopped fresh dill	5 mL
10	sheets filo pastry	10
I cup	melted butter	240 mL

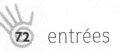 cook's tip

Uncooked spanakopita freeze beautifully. Freeze them on a cookie sheet and place directly into the oven for a quick and decadent meal. To re-crisp leftover spanakopita, simply reheat them in the oven at 350°F for 20 minutes.

1. Coarsely chop the spinach or chard and steam just until it is wilted. Place it in a colander and press out the excess water.

2. In a medium-sized frying pan, sauté the onions, garlic, oregano and pepper in oil until the onions are transparent.

3. In a large bowl, combine the sautéed mixture with the steamed greens and the remaining ingredients.

4. Preheat the oven to 350°F. Using sharp scissors cut the filo sheets in half lengthways and place them all in one pile. Use a pastry brush to brush the top piece of pastry lightly with melted butter. Place about ¾ cup of the filling in the bottom right hand corner. Use your hands to lift the bottom edges of 2 sheets of filo and fold over and up to the left side edge making a triangle pocket with the filling inside. Continue this motion up the strip of these sheets of pastry, keeping your filling in this tight triangle pocket and brushing each side with butter before folding. When done, seal the pastry by brushing the entire pocket with butter, and place it on a baking sheet. Continue this until you've finished all 10 pockets and bake for 45-55 minutes, until each pastry is golden and bubbly.

— Moreka Jolar

Spinach Mushroom Enchiladas with Monterey Jack

The spinach and mushrooms make these enchiladas packed with nutritional vegetable goodness. A cup of toasted and chopped almonds or whole toasted sunflower seeds added to the filling provides a nutty crunch. A half cup of chopped fresh cilantro in the mix gives the dish a traditional and fragrant taste.

Preheat the oven to 350°F.

1. In a deep saucepan, sauté the onions, garlic, bell peppers, chili and salt in the oil until tender. Stir in the mushrooms and spinach and cook until most of the moisture evaporates and the spinach has wilted. Remove from heat and stir in ½ cup of the cheese.

2. Divide the mixture evenly into 6-8 tortillas. Roll up and lay into a lightly oiled baking dish. If using corn tortillas, top each enchilada with Mexican Red Sauce immediately after rolling so they don't split. Top with enchilada sauce and the remaining cup of cheese. Bake until bubbly and golden, approximately 45 minutes.

— *Moreka Jolar*

Serves 6-8

3 tbsp	sunflower or safflower oil	45 mL
1 cup	chopped yellow onions	240 mL
1 tbsp	crushed garlic	15 mL
4 cups	diced red bell peppers	960 mL
1 tsp	red chili flakes	5 mL
½ tsp	salt	2.5 mL
2 cups	sliced mushrooms	480 mL
7 oz.	fresh spinach coarsely chopped	200 g
1½ cup	grated Monterey Jack cheese	360 mL
3 cups	Mexican Red Sauce (page 103)	720 mL
6-8	corn or small flour tortillas	6-8

Sweet Potato and Chard Curry

Served immediately, the chard will hold its vibrant green color, offering a beautiful
contrast to the rich orange of the sweet potato. To make this part of an Indian feast,
serve it with Dal (page 36), Vegetable Korma (page 78) and baked pappadums.
Pappadums are thin, sometimes spicy, lentil crackers that are
usually fried in vegetable oil.

Serves 5-6

3 tbsp	sunflower or safflower oil	45 mL
3 cups	diced onions	720 mL
1	minced jalapeño*	1
1 tbsp	crushed garlic	15 mL
1 tbsp	freshly grated ginger	15 mL
2 tbsp	Fresh Curry Paste or Madras curry powder	30 mL
6 cups	cubed sweet potatoes with peel or 8 cups ½-inch cubed eggplant	1.4 L
5 cups	chopped chard leaves	1.2 L
	salt to taste	
	juice of 1 lemon	

1. In a deep saucepan, sauté the onions, jalapeño, garlic and ginger in the oil until the onions are transparent. Stir in the curry paste (page 107) or powder and sweet potatoes, reduce the heat and cover to allow the sweet potatoes to simmer until they are very soft, stirring them often to avoid sticking. When the sweet potato is cooked, stir in the chard, 2 cups at a time, and cover again, just until the chopped chard has wilted. This will only take a few minutes. Season with salt to taste and add the lemon juice right before serving.

* If you leave the seeds in the jalapeño the dish will be hotter.

— *Moreka Jolar*

 cook's tip

Uncooked pappadums can be found in specialty food shops. Here is an easy and light oven-baked variation on deep-fried pappadums. Heat the oven to 450° F. Using metal tongs, place the pappadums directly on the oven rack. Cook for 2 minutes or until the pappadum begins to bubble, but not brown. They may be a bit soft when you remove them, but they will become crispy in seconds.

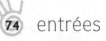

Thai Peanut Tofu

This long-time favorite of Hollyhock guests pairs tofu with chewy shiitake mushrooms in a long baking process which infuses the tofu with rich flavor. Garnish with toasted peanuts and offer a dish of crunchy won ton chips on the side. Serve over black Thai rice (see cook's tip) with Thai Curry Sauce (page 106).

1. In a large bowl, cover the dried mushrooms with boiling water. Cover and allow them to soak for 45 minutes. Drain off the water and thinly slice the mushrooms. Set aside.

2. Preheat the oven to 400°F. Blend all of the sauce ingredients in a food processor or blender just until mixed, approximately 30 seconds. This will help keep some of the crunch in the peanut butter.

3. In a large bowl, toss the sliced mushrooms with the tofu and cover them completely with peanut sauce. Mix well to ensure the sauce completely coats the tofu and mushrooms. Transfer to a well-oiled baking dish and place in the oven. Bake for approximately 1 hour, stirring every 20 minutes, until the tofu becomes evenly browned and a bit crunchy.

WON TON CHIPS

Won Ton chips are an excellent crunchy side dish to accompany Thai Peanut Tofu. Purchase 1 package of fresh won ton wrappers. Heat 2 inches of sunflower or safflower oil in a deep frying pan until very hot and fry each won ton wrapper until it is brown and crispy. Allow them to drain on paper towels.

— Moreka Jolar

Serves 6-8

3 cups	dry shiitake mushrooms	720 mL
25 oz.	firm tofu, cut into ½-inch-thick triangle pieces	715 g

SAUCE

1 cup	crunchy peanut butter or almond butter if you prefer	240 mL
½ cup	sunflower or safflower oil	120 mL
½ cup	tamari	120 mL
⅓ cup	fresh lemon juice	80 mL
3 tsp	crushed garlic	15 mL
3 tbsp	freshly grated ginger	45 mL
1	finely ground jalapeño	1

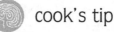

cook's tip

Black Thai rice, or purple rice, can be found in most specialty food stores. Rinse 1½ cups of black rice well and cook it with 2 cups water. In a saucepan, bring the rice and water to a boil, reduce heat to low, cover and continue to simmer until all the water has evaporated, approximately 30 minutes.

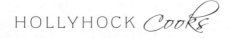

Torta Rustica

This is a homey Italian pie with a comforting taste. Save this for a day when you feel like spending a couple of hours in the kitchen. The end result is impressively delicious.

Serves 6-8

DOUGH

½ cup	warm water	120 mL
1 tsp	honey	5 mL
1 tbsp	active dry yeast	15 mL
1 cup	warm milk or soy milk	240 mL
1½ tsp	salt	7.5 mL
2 cups	whole wheat flour	480 mL
3 cups	unbleached white flour	960 mL

FILLING

2 tbsp	olive oil	30 mL
2 cups	chopped and rinsed leeks	480 mL
6 cups	coarsely chopped spinach, chard, kale, or young nettle leaves	1.4 L
½ cup	grated carrots	120 mL
¼ tsp	grated nutmeg	1.2 mL
1 tsp	black pepper	5 mL
2 tsp	chopped fresh basil	10 mL
¼ cup	chopped fresh parsley	1.2 mL
1 cup	grated Parmesan	240 mL
1 cup	cottage cheese or crumbled tofu	240 mL
1	egg	1

DOUGH

1. In a large bowl, dissolve the honey in the warm water and then sprinkle the yeast over this and let it stand for 10 minutes or until the yeast bubbles. Add the milk and salt and use a wooden spoon to stir in the whole wheat flour. Work in the remaining unbleached white flour until you can work the dough with your hands and then transfer it to a lightly floured surface and knead for 5 minutes. The dough should remain sticky. Shape the dough into a ball and set it in a warm spot in a covered bowl until doubled in bulk. This will take approximately 1 hour.

FILLING

2. In a large frying pan, sauté the leeks in the olive oil until tender. Toss in the greens of choice with the carrots, spices and herbs and continue to sauté until the greens reduce and some of the moisture evaporates. Set aside to cool slightly.

3. In a small bowl, whisk together the 2 cheeses with the egg. When the vegetables have cooled slightly, combine all these filling ingredients together in a large bowl.

ASSEMBLY

4. Preheat the oven to 350°F. Punch down the dough and cut it in half. Use a rolling pin to roll out half of the dough quite thinly on a lightly oiled surface until it is just a bit bigger than the diameter of a 9-inch pie dish. Press the dough into the dish and trim the edges to fit. Pour in the filling.

5. Roll out the remaining dough and cut it in to strips 1 inch in width. Weave these, lattice fashion, over the pie and pinch where the pieces join the bottom crust at the edge. Bake for 30-45 minutes. The top should be really well browned. Serve warm or at room temperature.

— *Moreka Jolar*

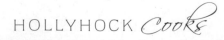

Vegetable Curry with Chickpeas

This curry served on a bed of rice is a meal on its own. It has a rich and creamy coconut sauce and the chickpeas provide a lot of protein. The difference between using a curry paste that's been sitting in the store for a year and making your own from mixed seeds and fresh herbs ground into a paste is palatable. It will lift this dish out of the realm of the merely delicious into the rarefied world of the simply divine.

1. In a deep saucepan, sauté the onions in butter or oil until they are tender. Add the carrots and continue to cook for another 10 minutes, stirring often. Add the zucchini and green beans and cook until the zucchini begins to soften. Add the bell peppers and chickpeas and continue to cook gently.

2. In a small bowl, whisk the curry paste thoroughly into the coconut milk and stir it into the vegetable mixture. Reduce the heat and continue to cook until all is tender, approximately 20 minutes. Be careful not to allow the coconut milk to boil. Season with salt to taste and serve on its own or over a bed of saffron rice (page 85).

VARIATIONS

Just before serving try adding one or more of the following:

- ⅓ cup packed fresh cilantro
- 1 cup whole toasted cashews
- 2 cups cubed fresh tomatoes
- 3 cups packed chopped kale or mustard greens

— *Moreka Jolar*

Serves 6-8

¼ cup	butter or sunflower or safflower oil	60 mL
2 cups	diced onions	480 mL
2 cups	carrots cut in coarse rounds	480 mL
4 cups	green or yellow zucchini cut in large cubes	960 mL
1 cup	halved green beans	240 mL
2 cups	assorted bell peppers coarsely chopped	480 mL
2 cups	cooked chickpeas	480 mL
2 cups	coconut milk	480 mL
⅓ cup	Fresh Curry Paste (page 107)	80 mL
	salt to taste	

 cook's tip

If you are using uncooked chickpeas, cover 1 cup of dry chickpeas generously with water and allow them to soak overnight. The next day, add 2 bay leaves and a small handful of coriander seeds to the water and bring it to a rolling boil. The coriander seeds make the chickpeas easier to digest. Continue to boil until the chickpeas are tender. This can take up to 3 hours, so you may need to add more water. Organic beans tend to take a little bit longer.

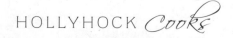

Vegetable Korma

Colorful and bold in flavor, Hollyhock's korma has a very fragrant and enticing aroma.
This multi-cultural fusion of island and India acquires more flavor when
served the next day so the cardamom, cloves and cinnamon
have time to thoroughly permeate the sauce.

Serves 6-8

3 tbsp	butter or sunflower or safflower oil	45 mL
3 cups	finely sliced onions	720 mL
2	fresh seeded and minced jalapeños	2
¼ cup	freshly shredded ginger	60 mL
2 tbsp	crushed garlic	30 mL
2 tsp	turmeric	10 mL
1 tsp	whole cardamom seeds	5 mL
5-8	whole cloves	5-8
1	large cinnamon stick	1
2	bay leaves	2
1 tsp	ground coriander	5 mL
1	cauliflower cut in flowerets	1
2 cups	coarsely chopped bite-sized carrots	480 mL
2 cups	chopped red bell pepper	480 mL
1 cup	chopped green bell pepper	240 mL
1 cup	chopped green beans	240 mL
2 cups	yogurt	480 mL
3 cups	coconut milk	720 mL
	salt to taste	
1 cup	chopped fresh cilantro	240 mL

1. In a large saucepan, sauté the onions, jalapeño, ginger and garlic in the oil or butter until the onions are transparent. Add the remaining whole and ground spices and continue to cook on low heat for another 5-10 minutes. Add the cauliflower and carrots and continue to cook on medium heat until the cauliflower is just beginning to get tender. Add the bell peppers, beans, yogurt and coconut milk, reduce the heat and continue to cook on low heat until all the vegetables are tender. Season with salt to taste and garnish with cilantro. Serve it over rice.

VARIATIONS
For added protein, mix in 1 block of firm, diced tofu with the peppers and beans. Add a couple of handfuls of roasted cashews, if desired. For a non-dairy version of this dish, replace the yogurt with 2 cups of coconut milk.

— *Moreka Jolar*

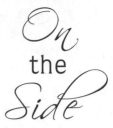

On the Side

INVENTIVE PREPARATIONS OF VEGETABLES and seafood infused with flavors from all over the world appear nightly on the Hollyhock dinner table. Here is a mouth-watering array of recipes for side dishes that are great complements to delicious entrées. Gravies, salsas and chutneys offer endless possibilities to experiment with new combinations of taste and color and foods from various cultures. Unique and original serving suggestions for dishes, such as Banana Chutney, which can be served at an Indian feast with samosas or over oatmeal, or cold cereal for breakfast, offer further inspiration. New twists on old favorites like Mashed Potatoes with Roasted Garlic and Chives or our Antipasto Platter offer surprising perspectives and flavors.

Every night at dinner, the Hollyhock cooks include one or two delectable dishes to compliment and augment the taste, color and consistency of the entrée. Although we serve them as side dishes, many of the following recipes can easily become the cornerstone of a light and satisfying meal, especially when served with bread, over a steaming bowl of pasta or with rice. Serve a sampling of three or four selections from our array of fabulous side dishes for a unique dinner party menu or family meal.

At Hollyhock, our side dishes are flavorful, out of the ordinary, and richly textured little feasts. Here are some simple, exciting, edible ideas to add spirit and soul to the heart of your meal.

FOUR

Antipasto Platter

Antipasto is an Italian word that means "before the meal." Antipasti are appetizers that are generally served cold. These oven-roasted carrots and asparagus are naturally sweet and full-bodied. The simple tomato and parsley salad is a palate cleanser. Arrange each of these antipasti in three separate piles on one large platter or, if you like, on a bed of greens. Top them with marinated artichoke hearts, cubed cheese such as feta, and your favorite olives. Barbecued mushrooms (page 83) and roasted fennel with dill (page 85) make great additions to the platter.

Serves 6-8

PEPPERED CARROTS

4 cups	julienned carrots	960 mL
2 tbsp	olive oil	30 mL
1 tbsp	balsamic vinegar	15 mL
2 tsp	fresh coarse cracked pepper	10 mL

GARLIC-ROASTED ASPARAGUS

6 cups or 2 bunches	asparagus	1.4 L
2 tbsp	olive oil	30 mL
3 tsp	crushed garlic	15 mL
¼ tsp	salt	1.2 mL

TOMATO AND PARSLEY

4 cups	tomato wedges	960 mL
3 tbsp	chopped fresh parsley	45 mL
1 tbsp	balsamic vinegar	15 mL
	salt and pepper to taste	

Preheat the oven to 450°F.

PEPPERED CARROTS

1. Combine all the ingredients and spread them out on a baking sheet and bake for 30-45 minutes, until tender. Cool.

GARLIC-ROASTED ASPARAGUS

1. Snap the tough ends off the asparagus spears (see cook's tip on page 84) and cut them in half crosswise.

2. Combine all the ingredients and spread them out on a baking sheet. Bake them at 450°F for 20 minutes, or until they turn a bright green. Cool.

TOMATO AND PARSLEY

1. Combine all the ingredients. Serve at room temperature.

— *Moreka Jolar*

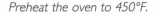

cook's tip

When you see the word "julienne" in a recipe, it means to cut a vegetable into long, thin, matchstick strips.

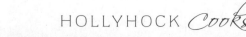

Acorn Squash with Orange and Nutmeg

Here we've slathered the small and firm winter squash in zesty orange and fragrant nutmeg. The long baking time reveals the natural sweetness in acorn squash and renders the thick skin tender. Garnish with chopped fresh parsley or cilantro, and orange slices.

Preheat the oven to 350°F.

1. Use a large, heavy knife or a cleaver to cut open the squash. Remove the seeds and cut the squash into 2-inch pieces, leaving the skin on.

2. In a small bowl, combine the orange juice, oil, orange zest, nutmeg and salt and whisk.

3. Toss the acorn squash with all the ingredients until it is well covered. Bake on a baking sheet for 1 hour or until it is tender.

— *Moreka Jolar*

Serves 6-8

2 lbs.	acorn squash	915 g
¼ cup	fresh orange juice	60 mL
2 tbsp	sunflower or safflower oil	30 mL
1 tbsp	orange zest	15 mL
½ tsp	freshly grated nutmeg	2.5 mL
¼ tsp	salt	1.2 mL
1 tsp	chili flakes, if desired	5 mL

Baby Bok Choy with Mushrooms and Whole Toasted Almonds

Here is a classic Chinese combination. Fresh young bok choy greens and crunchy nuts are mixed with tender, meaty mouthfuls of mushrooms. Serve it as a side with an Asian dinner.

1. In a large wok, cook the mushrooms on medium heat with the oil. Toss them around until they begin to brown, approximately 10 minutes. Reduce the heat and cover. As the mushrooms cook, all the water will come out of them and give them a good steaming. Cook for another 10 minutes. Add the bok choy, cover and steam for 2 minutes.

2. Combine the water, tamari, cornstarch and garlic in a bowl and whisk until the cornstarch is dissolved. Add this to the mushrooms and bok choy and bring heat up a bit. Allow it to cook with the lid off as the sauce thickens. Stir to cover the vegetables with the thick sauce. Pour it onto a serving platter and garnish with whole almonds. Serve hot.

— *Moreka Jolar*

Serves 8-10

3 tbsp	sunflower or safflower oil	45 mL
12 cups	packed coarsely chopped baby bok choy	3 L
12 cups	packed small whole mushrooms	3 L
¼ cup	water	60 mL
¼ cup	tamari	60 mL
1 tbsp	corn starch	15 mL
2 tsp	minced garlic	10 mL
½ cup	whole toasted almonds	120 mL

 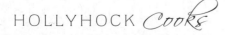

Baked Beans with Epazote

Epazote is a commonly used green leafy herb, native to Mexico, and it gives baked beans an authentic Mexican flavor. Serve this hearty dish with Spinach Mushroom Enchiladas with Monterey Jack (page 73) or as a dip.

Serves 6-8

5 cups	cooked beans, such as kidney, pinto or black turtle beans	1.2 L
3 cups	water	720 mL
2 cups	diced onions	480 mL
⅓ cup	oil	80 mL
1 tbsp	minced garlic	15 mL
2 tsp	epazote *	10 mL
2 tsp	ancho chili powder	10 mL
1 tsp	salt	5 mL

Preheat the oven to 350°F.

1. Combine the ingredients in a well-oiled casserole dish. Bake for 2 hours, stirring every half hour. Mash lightly with a potato masher, or leave as is, and serve beside enchiladas with salsa, or serve as a dip.

* Epazote is available in specialty food stores. Check it for large twigs before adding.

— *Moreka Jolar*

cook's tip

If you use dry beans in this hearty recipe with Mexican overtones, soak 2½ cups of beans in plenty of water overnight. Bring the beans to a boil the next morning with a couple of bay leaves and cook them in lots of water until tender. Cooking time will vary according to the type of bean. Organic beans can take as long as 4 hours or more.

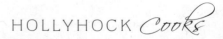

Barbecued Mushrooms

This is a succulent and simple way to prepare fresh mushrooms. Slowly cooking them on the barbecue turns them into tender, juicy morsels. If you are using small mushrooms, such as white mushrooms, it may be necessary to use a perforated barbecue basket or another metal tray with small holes in it to ensure the mushrooms do not fall through the grill.

Preheat the barbecue on low.

1. In a large bowl, toss the mushrooms with the oil and salt. This will look like a lot of food but the mushrooms will really reduce after cooking.

2. Put the mushrooms into a perforated barbecue basket. Grill the mushrooms for about 30-45 minutes, turning them often until the mushrooms are brown and tender. Serve immediately, or at room temperature, as a part of the Antipasto Platter (page 80).

— *Hanyu Wasyliw*

Serves 2-4

1 lb.	whole mushrooms	460 g
½ cup	olive oil	120 mL
¼ cup	coarse sea salt	60 mL

Bell Peppers Stuffed with Cherry Tomatoes

This is another visually beautiful dish. Serve it as a starter with crusty bread to soak up the sweet juices or beside your favorite pasta dish. The process of baking or oven-roasting vegetables brings out all the natural sugars present in fresh foods. This is especially evident with sweet peppers and tomatoes.

Preheat the oven to 350°F.

1. Cut the bell peppers in half lengthwise, through the stalk, keeping the stalk intact. This helps hold them together while baking. Remove the seeds and the pith from the peppers.

2. Place the peppers in a baking dish and fill with them with cherry tomatoes, approximately 10 halves per pepper but this will vary depending on size. Drizzle 1 tbsp of olive oil and 1 tsp honey over the tomatoes in each pepper. Add a pinch of salt and pepper. Bake for 40 minutes or until the peppers have wilted and are browning in some spots. Serve warm.

— *Annabel Davis*

Serves 6

3	medium-sized red or yellow bell peppers	3
2 cups	halved cherry tomatoes	480 mL
6 tbsp	olive oil	90 mL
6 tsp	honey	30 mL
	salt and pepper to taste	

 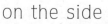

Carrot and Asparagus Sesame Stir-fry

Cook this vibrant, colorful stir-fry hot and fast so the carrot and asparagus get roasted,
while retaining their crunch. Serve it over rice and with Thai Peanut Tofu (page 75).

Serves 6-8

6 cups	carrots, thinly and diagonally sliced	1.4 L
6 cups	fresh asparagus, ends snapped off and cut in two	1.4 L
⅓ cup	tamari	80 mL
3 tbsp	grated fresh ginger	45 mL
⅓ cup	toasted sesame seeds	80 mL

cook's tip

Here's how to prepare asparagus: Since fresh asparagus has tough ends, the best way to get off all the tough part is to snap it, rather than cut it. When you snap the ends off, they'll break right at the point of tenderness. What remains will be fit for royalty.

1. Heat a small amount of sesame oil in a hot wok and cook the carrots, stirring constantly until they begin to brown, for approximately 2 minutes. Add the asparagus spears. Keep the heat on high and continue stirring. Continue to cook just until the asparagus begins to turn a bright green color and is tender when pierced with a fork.

2. Reduce the heat and add the tamari and fresh ginger. Stir just until the vegetables are covered with sauce. Remove from the heat and toss in the toasted seeds.

— *Moreka Jolar*

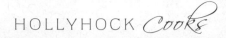

Fennel and Carrot Roast
with Fresh Dill

The mild and rustic tastes of roasted fennel and carrots are mellow and sweet.
Serve this very easy dish hot beside Nut Loaf (page 63) or pasta, or add it to the
Antipasto Platter (page 80) at room temperature.

Preheat the oven to 350°F.

1. In a large bowl, toss the fennel and carrots with all the remaining ingredients. Spread them out on a baking sheet and bake for approximately 1 hour, until the fennel and carrots are browned and tender.

— *Moreka Jolar*

Serves 6-8

4 cups	fresh fennel bulb, cut in large slices	960 mL
4 cups	carrots, sliced thickly and diagonally	960 mL
¼ cup	olive oil	60 mL
¼ cup	white wine vinegar	60 mL
2 tbsp	chopped fresh dill	30 mL
1 tbsp	minced garlic	15 mL
½ tsp	salt	2.5 mL

Fragrant Saffron Rice

Exotic saffron strands come from a kind of crocus flower native to Asia and parts of Europe.
The boiling water allows the saffron to release its red color and subtle taste. This delicately
flavored rice is an excellent addition to any Indian feast and works well as a side
to Vegetable Korma (page 78) or Sweet Potato and Chard Curry (page 74).

1. In a small bowl, pour the ½ cup of boiling water over the saffron and allow it to sit for 10 minutes.

2. In a small, heavy saucepan, combine the saffron and water with the rice, ¾ cup of water, cardamom and cloves. Cover and bring to a boil. Reduce the heat to low and simmer until all the water has gone and the rice is tender. Fluff with a fork and serve hot.

— *Moreka Jolar*

Serves 3-4

1 pinch	saffron strands	1
½ cup	boiling water	120 mL
2 cups	jasmine rice	480 mL
¾ cup	water	180 mL
½ tsp	cardamom seeds	2.5 mL
4	whole cloves	4

Garlic Potato Gratin with Chèvre

It is a bit of a process to prepare this smooth gratin, but the end result is well worth the effort.
This dish is creamy, elegant and luxurious, with a hint of nutmeg.

Serves 6-8

3 lbs.	potatoes	1.4 kg
6	whole cloves garlic	6
4¼ cups	whole milk	1 L
1	bouquet garni *	1
	freshly grated nutmeg to taste	
	salt to taste	
2 tbsp	butter	30 mL
1 cup	heavy cream	240 mL
8 oz.	chèvre	230 g
	freshly ground pepper to taste	

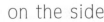 cook's tip

Although we prefer the taste and texture of Yukon Gold or other yellow-fleshed potatoes, this dish is also delicious made with red or baking potato varieties. There is no need to peel Yukon Gold or red potatoes but you may want to peel russet or baking potatoes.

Preheat the oven to 375°F.

1. Scrub the potatoes well and thinly slice them into whole rounds. Lightly smash the garlic cloves with the flat of a knife, but do not chop.

2. In a large, heavy-bottomed saucepan, combine the potatoes and garlic cloves with the milk, bouquet garni, nutmeg, salt and butter. Bring to a boil over moderately high heat, stirring occasionally to prevent the potatoes from sticking. Reduce the heat and simmer, stirring approximately 10 to 15 minutes depending on the variety of potato and how thinly they are sliced. Remove from heat when they are just beginning to be tender but not crumbling.

3. Use a slotted spoon to transfer the potatoes and garlic to a buttered 9x13-inch baking dish discarding the bouquet garni and milk. Pour the heavy cream over the potatoes and sprinkle with additional nutmeg and pepper, and top with crumbled chèvre. Place in the middle of the oven and bake approximately 1 hour, until crisp and golden on the top. If the top is browning too quickly, before the potatoes are done, cover the dish lightly with foil.

VARIATIONS

For a more traditional gratin, use 2 cups coarsely grated Gruyère, Swiss or aged white cheddar. Mix the grated cheese with the heavy cream. Layer the potato mixture with the cheese mixture in the baking dish, topping it off with cheese.

* Bouquet garni can be made of sprigs of fresh parsley, fresh thyme and 1 bay leaf, all tied together with kitchen twine.

— *Hanyu Wasyliw*

 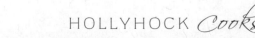

Oysters

The shoreline of Cortes Island is rich with fresh oysters and the weekly oyster barbecue on the beach at Hollyhock celebrates this delicate shellfish. We serve oysters on the half shell over a seaside grill or fire pit with Hollyhock Oyster Barbecue Sauce (page 102). Here are a few more ideas for preparing fresh oysters.

OYSTERS ON THE HALF SHELL WITH SAUCE

Prepare them on the half shell with a spoonful of Roasted Red Pepper Sauce (pg 104) and/or Cilantro Pesto with Sesame and Lime (page 113) and place the oysters under the broiler until done the way you like them.

— *Rowan Brooks*

OYSTERS ON THE HALF SHELL WITH CRISPY FRIED CAPERS

Bake or broil the oysters on the half shell and garnish them with lime juice, fresh cilantro leaves and crispy fried capers.

— *Linda Gardner*

BREADED OYSTERS PAN-FRIED IN HERB BUTTER

Roll the raw oysters in flour then dip them in a mix of equal portions of egg and milk. Coat them with breadcrumbs and pan-fry in Herb Butter for Seafood (page 117).

— *Jenica Rayne*

Green Beans Indian Style

After the traditional Indian spices are infused in hot oil, the beans are added and cooked to perfection. This dish is easy to prepare and classic in taste. Serve it with Vegetable Curry with Chickpeas (page 77) and Fragrant Saffron Rice (page 85).

Serves 6-8

½ cup	olive oil	120 mL
I tbsp	turmeric	15 mL
2 tbsp	whole cumin seeds	30 mL
2 tbsp	whole mustard seeds	30 mL
I tsp	cayenne	5 mL
½ tsp	salt	2.5 mL
8-10 cups	green beans, cut lengthwise	2-2.5 L

1. In a large frying pan, heat the oil and all the spices and seeds and stir until they start to pop. Add the beans and stir to coat with the oil and spices, lower the heat and cover to simmer for 10 minutes. Stir every so often until the beans are tender. Serve immediately.

— *Rosemary Wooldridge*

" I used to be a visual artist and what I love best about Hollyhock's food is the colorfulness and the beauty of the presentation".
— Sharon Butala

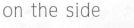

Mashed Potatoes with Roasted Garlic and Chives

Mashed potatoes are the ultimate comforting pleasure food. Here's a new, silky-textured twist on an old favorite. Serve these mashed potatoes beside just about anything, including Nut Loaf (page 63) with Nut Butter Gravy or Miso Gravy (page 100).

1. Peel the potatoes, if you like, and cut them into large sections. Cover the potatoes generously with water in a large pot and boil until they are tender, about 20-25 minutes. Drain the water and return the potatoes to the pot.

2. In a small frying pan, roast the whole garlic cloves in oil until they are well browned on all sides. Add the garlic cloves, including the oil from the frying pan, with the butter, milk, salt, pepper and chives to the potatoes and mash them well with a potato masher.

— *Moreka Jolar*

8-10 servings

2½ lbs. or 6	medium-sized baking potatoes	1.1 kg or 6
10	cloves of garlic	10
¼ cup	butter	60 mL
½ cup	milk	120 mL
1 tsp	salt	5 mL
1 tsp	black pepper	5 mL
2 tbsp	chopped fresh chives	30 mL

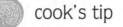 cook's tip

To avoid gluey mashed potatoes, always use baking potatoes and not red or new potatoes. Baking potatoes have less moisture and will remain light and fluffy.

 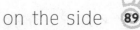

Pattypan Squash with Yogurt-Hazelnut Sauce

Pattypan is a very tender and mild squash, though any tender summer squash will do in its place. The creamy yogurt-hazelnut sauce is the perfect nutty and mellow topping.

Serves 6-8

3 lbs. or 5	large pattypan squash	1.4 kg or 5
1½ cups	yogurt	360 mL
¾ cup	toasted and ground hazelnuts	180 mL
2	minced shallots	2
1 tbsp	chopped fresh dill	15 mL
½ tsp	salt	2.5 mL
½ tsp	black pepper	2.5 mL

1. In a small bowl, combine the yogurt, hazelnuts, shallots, dill, salt and pepper and mix well with a whisk. Cut the squash into large 2-inch pieces and steam just until they are tender. Serve immediately, topped with the sauce.

— *Moreka Jolar*

Moroccan Baked Squash

This is a surprising and wonderful fusion of flavors. The thick skin of the winter squash is tender after the long baking process. The taste is bold and the Moroccan black olives are a pleasing, mild addition. Garnish with chili flakes, chopped walnuts, or bits of soft chèvre to create delightful variations. Serve hot beside fish or quiche.

Serves 6-8

6 cups or 2 lbs.	squash such as delicatta, butternut other winter squash cut in 2-inch pieces	1.4 L or 915g
¼ cup	olive oil	60 mL
¼ cup	fresh lemon juice	60 mL
1 tbsp	brown sugar	15 mL
1 tbsp	freshly grated ginger	15 mL
1 tsp	ground cumin	5 mL
1 tsp	ground coriander	5 mL
½ cup	dry-cured Moroccan black olives *	120 mL

Preheat the oven to 350°F.

1. In a large bowl, whisk together the oil, lemon juice, sugar, ginger, cumin and coriander. Add the squash and toss it all with your hands until it is well coated. Spread the squash out on a lightly oiled baking sheet and bake until tender and caramelized, about 45-50 minutes. Remove from the oven and toss in the olives before serving.

* Dry-cured Moroccan black olives are available in specialty foods delis. Other dry-cured olives will work as well.

— *Stephen Fosker*

Roasted Barley Pilaf with Mushrooms and Hazelnuts

Pilaf, and varied ethnic relatives such as pilau, is a slow-cooked dish traditionally made with rice. This Hollyhock twist is a rich, full side dish that can be served beside your favorite seafood entrée. Roasting the barley gives this pilaf a nutty taste. For a traditional and sweet taste, try adding dried currants or sliced apple. For additional variety, you can use almonds or pine nuts in place of the hazelnuts.

1. In a large frying pan, sauté the onions, mushrooms, peppers, garlic and thyme with the oil just until the peppers begin to get tender. Set aside.

2. In a large, heavy saucepan, dry toast the barley over low heat for approximately 15 to 20 minutes, stirring frequently, until it starts to brown and smell roasted. Add the water or broth, cover and allow to the dish to simmer until all the liquid has evaporated and the barley is tender, approximately 20-30 minutes. Mix in the sautéed vegetables and season with salt and pepper to taste. Toss in the nuts right before serving to ensure they keep their crunch. Serve garnished with chopped scallion.

— *Moreka Jolar*

Serves 6-8

1½ cups	pearl barley	360 mL
2 tbsp	olive oil	30 mL
2 cups	chopped onions	480 mL
2 cups	sliced mushrooms	480 mL
2 cups	diced red or yellow bell pepper	480 mL
2 tbsp	crushed garlic	30 mL
2 tsp	chopped fresh thyme	10 mL
3 cups	hot vegetable stock or water	720 mL
	salt and pepper to taste	
1 cup	toasted and chopped hazelnuts	240 mL
3	chopped scallions for garnish	3

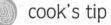 cook's tip

Dry toasting a grain, as explained in the above recipe, brings out the grain's unique flavor, resulting in a flaky and not mushy texture after it is cooked. Follow this procedure with rice, millet, quinoa, oats and others. Toasted grains need less water to cook, so keep this in mind when using them in any recipe.

 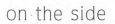

Roasted Roots with Lemon and Rosemary

You can leave the skin on all the roots you roast in this recipe. They will become very tender while baking and will be delicious to eat. Heat up the leftovers and serve them with morning eggs. Serve this dish garnished with lemon wedges and fresh rosemary sprigs beside Spanakopita (page 72), Hummus (page 110) and Tzatzki (page 95).

Serves 6-8

2 cups	yams, cut into 1-inch cubes	480 mL
2 cups	potatoes, cut into 1-inch cubes	480 mL
2 cups	beets, cut into 1-inch cubes	480 mL
2 cups	carrots, cut into large pieces	480 mL
2 cups	onions, cut into large pieces	480 mL
16	whole cloves garlic	16
½ cup	olive oil	120 mL
	juice of 2 lemons	
2 tbsp	minced garlic	30 mL
¼ cup	coarsely chopped fresh rosemary	60 mL
1 tsp	salt	5 mL
1 tsp	black pepper	5 mL

Preheat the oven to 400°F.

1. In a large bowl, toss all the vegetables with the olive oil, lemon juice, garlic, rosemary, salt and pepper. Spread them out on a baking sheet and roast for half an hour. Toss well with a spatula and roast for another half hour. Serve hot.

— *Moreka Jolar*

cook's tip

In the autumn, place colorful leaves around the serving dishes to add to the visual pleasure of a meal.

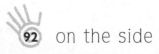

Three Easy Ways to Prepare Tofu

Tofu is like a giant sponge waiting to soak up flavors. These are just a few quick ways to prepare simple and delicious tofu. Serve warm beside steamed greens, in a stir-fry, or cold over a fresh green salad. Each recipe requires one block of firm tofu, approximately 360 grams.

YEASTED TOFU

1. Cut the tofu into half-inch cubes and sauté it in a non-stick frying pan with the oil until golden and crunchy, approximately 10 minutes. Stir often to brown all the sides.

2. Sprinkle the yeast over the tofu, reduce the heat, and stir until the tofu is well coated.

3. In a small bowl, combine the tamari and water and pour it over the tofu. Continue to cook on low and stir until the tofu is coated in a thick, gravy-like sauce. Serve hot with rice and steamed vegetables or cold over a salad.

— Rowan Brooks

SESAME BAKED TOFU

Preheat the oven to 375°F.

1. Cut the tofu into cubes and marinate it in a mixture of oil, soy sauce, sugar, garlic and ginger for at least 2 hours.

2. Combine the ground seeds with the flour in a small bowl.

3. Drain off the marinade and roll the tofu pieces in the mix of sesame seeds and flour. Lay the tofu on a lightly oiled baking sheet and bake for 20 minutes, turning the tofu over a few times to ensure it is brown on all sides. Serve hot or cold.

— Rosemary Wooldridge

GINGER-MISO TOFU

1. Cut the tofu into 2-inch pieces and marinate it in the Ginger-Miso Sauce for at least 2 hours. Cook it in a non-stick frying pan or bake it at 350°F until crispy. Serve hot or cold, garnished with scallions.

— Moreka Jolar

Serves 2

YEASTED TOFU

3 tbsp	olive, sunflower or safflower oil	45 mL
¼ cup	tamari	60 mL
¼ cup	water	60 mL
½ cup	nutritional flake yeast	120 mL

SESAME BAKED TOFU

2 tbsp	sunflower or safflower oil	30 mL
3 tbsp	soy sauce	45 mL
2 tsp	sugar	10 mL
1 tsp	minced fresh garlic	5 mL
1 tsp	minced ginger	5 mL
⅓ cup	toasted and ground sesame seeds	80 mL
3 tbsp	flour	45 mL

GINGER-MISO TOFU

1 cup	Ginger-MisoSauce (pg 102)	240 mL
1	chopped scallion to garnish	1

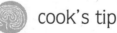 **cook's tip**

Toasted and ground pumpkin seeds and nori serve as a tasty and iron-rich topping for grains and vegetables. Dry toast the seeds in a small frying pan and then finely grind the seeds and nori in separate batches in a coffee or spice grinder. Store in a sealed container on the table to have available as a condiment at all meals.

Sesame Home Fries

These healthy baked fries make this favorite side dish a nutritious choice. Serve them at breakfast or with Nut Loaf (page 63) for supper. Cover them with Miso or Nut Butter Gravy (page 100) and they're practically an entrée on their own.

Serves 6

3 lbs.	potatoes	1.4 kg
2 tbsp	olive oil	30 mL
2 tbsp	sesame seeds	30 mL
2 tsp	ancho chili powder *	10 mL
1 tsp	turmeric, if desired	5 mL
1 tsp	salt	5 mL
½ tsp	pepper	2.5 mL

Preheat the oven to 400°F.

1. Cut the potatoes lengthways into ½-inch-thick wedges. Combine the oil with the remaining ingredients and toss this with the potatoes until the potatoes are totally covered.

2. Spread the potatoes out over a baking sheet and bake until they turn crispy on top, then turn the fries over and bake them again until crisp and browned, approximately 1½ hours in total.

* Ancho chili powder is known for its rich, full-bodied flavor and not its heat. It is available in specialty food stores.

— *Moreka Jolar*

Green Apple Raita

Raita is a classic, creamy and cooling side dish to a spicy Indian feast. This refreshing dish is traditionally made with cucumber. Here's a new, sweet, apple-sensation variation.

Makes 3 cups

1½ cups	grated firm green apples	360 mL
1½ cups	yogurt	360 mL
1 tsp	whole cumin seeds	5 mL
1 tsp	chopped fresh mint	5 mL
	salt to taste, if desired	

1. In a small bowl, combine the yogurt and the grated apple immediately so the apple doesn't turn brown. Set aside.

2. In a small, dry frying pan, toast the cumin seeds until they begin to brown. Add the seeds, mint and salt to the yogurt mixture. Mix. Chill and serve.

— *Moreka Jolar*

Tzatziki

Tzatziki is a classic creamy Middle Eastern dip or side dish. Lavished on fresh pitas (page 140) or set beside Roasted Roots with Lemon and Rosemary (page 92), this dish can make the meal. It can also be served over Tabouleh with Toasted Seeds (page 27) and stuffed into a pita pocket to make an excellent lunch.

1. Press the grated cucumber into a sieve or colander to remove the excess water. Mix well with the remaining ingredients and allow it to chill for 20 minutes before serving.

— Moreka Jolar

Makes 3 cups

1½ cups	grated cucumber	360 mL
2 cups	yogurt	480 mL
1 tbsp	crushed garlic	15 mL
1 tbsp	chopped fresh dill	15 mL
1 tsp	chopped fresh mint	5 mL
	salt to taste	

" It makes my body, heart and mind sing to eat the luscious food at Hollyhock and know that it was grown with care and without the chemicals that threaten the earth and our survival. It is sadly ironic that we live in a world today where the majority of food that is consumed to nourish our bodies contains toxic chemicals and has been grown in ways that contribute to the poisoning of our biosphere. If we are to nourish ourselves and heal the earth we need to start here, by meeting our basic needs with wholesome organic food. What a joy that Hollyhock helps us to do that while tempting our palette with delicious creations. "
— Tzeporah Berman

Guacamole

Guacamole is a spicy, creamy sauce or dip from Mexico, the avocado's homeland. It is a perfect partner to enchiladas and to salsa and tortilla chips. You can freshen it up and fill it out by mixing in a cup of freshly grated zucchini.

Makes 4 cups

4-5	ripe avocados or 3 cups (720 mL) mashed	4-5
	juice of 1 lime	
½ cup	diced tomato	120 mL
⅓ cup	finely diced purple onion	80 mL
1 tbsp	crushed garlic	15 mL
	salt and pepper to taste	
1-2 tbsp	chopped fresh cilantro, if desired	15-30 mL
1	seeded and diced jalapeño, if desired	1

1. In a medium-sized bowl, add the lime juice immediately to the avocados to prevent the avocado from turning brown. Mash them with a fork or a potato masher. Mix in all the remaining ingredients and season to taste. Cover the surface with more lime juice and plastic wrap until you are ready to serve.

— *Kira Kotilla*

 cook's tip

If you need to store guacamole for any length of time, add a couple of avocado pits to prevent the avocado from browning. Then cover the surface with more lime juice and place plastic wrap directly on the surface. Refrigerate and enjoy later.

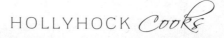

Mango Salsa

With the juicy sweetness of mango, this chunky salsa sizzles when served as an accompaniment to Mexican foods or as an appetizer with tortilla chips.

1. Combine the ingredients and refrigerate for 1 hour before serving. Include the jalapeño seeds if you want more heat.

* Salsa is best made with ripe, but firm, fruit. Over-ripe fruit will turn mushy. Four large mangoes will equal about 3½ cups diced.

— *Kira Kotilla*

Makes 4 cups

3½ cups	diced mango, pineapple or papaya *	840 mL
½ cup	finely diced purple onion	120 mL
½ cup	diced red bell pepper	120 mL
	juice of ½ lime	
2	seeded and minced jalapeño peppers	2
2 tbsp	chopped fresh cilantro	30 mL
	salt to taste	

Pico De Gallo Salsa

Cilantro is the basic flavor in this hot salsa. Chipotle peppers can be substituted for the jalapeño for a hot smoky flavor.

1. In a small bowl, combine all the ingredients and refrigerate for 1 hour before serving. If you want the salsa to be hotter include the jalapeño seeds.

— *Kira Kotilla*

Makes 5 cups

4 cups	diced fresh tomatoes	960 mL
¾ cup	diced purple onions	180 mL
1 tbsp	crushed garlic	15 mL
¼ cup	chopped fresh cilantro	60 mL
2	seeded and minced jalapeño peppers	2
	juice of 1 lime	
	salt and pepper to taste	

Banana Chutney

Sweet and bursting with ginger and lime and with a hint of cloves, this chutney is very easy and versatile. It is a must with samosas or an Indian feast, but is also delicious at breakfast, served over oatmeal or cold cereal.

Makes 3 cups

8	large bananas	8
2 tbsp	freshly grated ginger	30 mL
	juice of ½ lime	
5	whole cloves	5
1 tsp	chili flakes, if desired	5 mL

1. Mash the bananas with a fork. Combine all the ingredients in a non-stick frying pan and sauté for approximately 15 minutes, or until bubbly and hot. Transfer the entire mixture to a small bowl and cover the surface with plastic wrap. Refrigerate for at least 2 hours before serving.

— *Moreka Jolar*

Cashew Chutney

A thick texture and full-bodied flavor distinguishes this chutney from others. It has a strong and bold taste that is exotic and surprising. Serve it with Green Apple Raita (page 94) as a part of an Indian feast, or spread it on toast.

Makes 2 cups

⅔ cup	yellow split peas	160 mL
½ tbsp	whole fennel seeds	8 mL
1 cup	cashew nuts	240 mL
2 tbsp	freshly grated ginger	30 mL
1	seeded and minced green chili	1
⅓ cup	chopped fresh cilantro	80 mL
	salt to taste	

1. In a large, non-stick frying pan, dry toast the split peas, fennel seeds and cashews until they are browned in a few places. Add enough water to generously cover the ingredients and bring them to a boil for 3 minutes. Drain off the water.

2. Transfer the ingredients from the frying pan to a food processor and pulse until well chopped. Add the ginger, chili and cilantro, and pulse again. Slowly add water until the chutney reaches a desired consistency. Season with salt and chill until serving.

— *Dianne West*

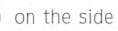
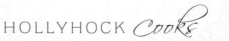

Coconut Cilantro Chutney

The vibrant, sweet crunch of coconut perfectly complements the tang of lime and fragrant cilantro. Cilantro lovers, dig your spoons into this thick and meaty chutney.

1. If using dried coconut, cover it with hot water and allow it to soak for 30 minutes. Strain off the water.

2. Place all the ingredients in a food processor or blender and blend until they have reached a desired consistency. Add more water or lime juice if desired. Serve chilled.

— *Moreka Jolar*

Makes 2 cups

2 cups	fresh or dry shredded coconut	480 mL
	zest and juice of 2 limes	
½	minced jalapeño pepper	½
1 cup	chopped fresh cilantro	240 mL
2 tbsp	freshly grated ginger	30 mL
2 tsp	crushed garlic	10 mL
	salt to taste	

Mango Chutney

Chutneys are an Indian tradition and no meal is complete without them. They enliven curries, giving a pleasing contrast of taste and flavor. Mango chutney is a classic that makes any dish a swanky partner, but it's particularly appealing with samosas or an Indian feast. It also is excellent served with fish. Mango can be mixed with sliced apples or pears if you like, or throw in some diced red bell pepper for a color contrast.

1. Combine all the ingredients and cook them in a saucepan on medium heat. Allow them to simmer for 30 minutes. Remove and chill in the refrigerator.

— *Rowan Brooks*

Makes 4 cups

4 cups	roughly chopped mango or 4 mangoes	960 mL
2 tbsp	freshly grated ginger	30 mL
3 tbsp	crushed garlic	45 mL
½ cup	apple cider vinegar	120 mL
1 tsp	hot red chili pepper minced or ½ tsp dry flakes	5 mL
	salt to taste	

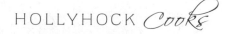

Miso Gravy

You'll never miss meat gravy again! This easy-to-prepare gravy is thick and rich with a bold flavor. Miso gravy makes just about anything it tops something to savor. Serve it hot over Nut Loaf (page 63), mashed potatoes, fries (page 89 & 94) or steamed vegetables. It keeps refrigerated for up to two weeks.

Makes 3 cups

½ cup	miso paste	120 mL
½ cup	sunflower or safflower oil	120 mL
3 tbsp	cornstarch	45 mL
2 tbsp	freshly grated ginger	30 mL
2 tsp	crushed garlic	10 mL
1 tsp	ground chili	5 mL
2 cups	water	480 mL

1. Mix all the ingredients except the water in a blender or food processor to form a paste. Then add the water and continue mixing. Transfer the mixture to a saucepan and heat on low. Use a wooden spoon to stir until the gravy has thickened. Whisk it if it gets lumpy.

— *Moreka Jolar*

Nut Butter Gravy

Serve this decadent, nutty and intensely flavored gravy over mashed potatoes (page 89), Nut Loaf (page 63) or Sesame Home Fries (page 94).

Makes 2 cups

1 cup	finely diced onions	240 mL
2 cups	diced mushrooms	480 mL
½ tsp	black pepper	2.5 mL
	pinch of chopped fresh marjoram	
1 cup	water	240 mL
⅔ cup	almond, hazelnut or cashew nut butter	160 mL
2 tbsp	tamari	30 mL

1. In a large frying pan, sauté the onions, mushrooms, black pepper and marjoram until the mushrooms are tender, approximately 10 minutes.

2. In a small bowl, whisk together the water, nut butter and tamari.

3. Remove the mushrooms from the heat and stir in the nut butter mixture. Place it back on low heat and simmer to thicken if desired. Be careful not to allow the gravy to get too hot or the nut butter will separate.

— *Rowan Brooks*

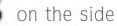

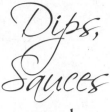

FIVE

Dips,
Sauces
and
Pâtés

LET'S STOP FOR A MOMENT and appreciate the smaller dishes. Dips, sauces and pâtés give a meal unexpected tastes and flavors. Protein-rich spreads make new and exciting sandwich fillings. Additions of nuts, flowers, herbs and spices turn ordinary blocks of butter into gourmet spreads. Sauces such as Mexican Red Sauce provide the final bold and fiery topping for Central American dishes. Pestos such as Cilantro Pesto with Sesame and Lime transform a bowl of pasta into a tangy, full-bodied, intensely flavored treat. Marinades like Ginger-Miso Sauce infuse fish or tofu with herbs and spices. Dips like Hot Artichoke Dip make a succulent accompaniment to crackers. Here you will find Hollyhock's Barbecue Sauce, made famous by our weekly beachside oyster barbecues during the summer. Explore this selection from the Hollyhock kitchen. These small dishes may be just the right touch to help a meal reach its full potential.

Ginger-Miso Sauce

Use this thick, tangy and spicy sauce over Soba Noodles with Ginger-Miso Eggplant (page 69) or as a marinade for fish or tofu. The recipe calls for mirin, a sweetened rice vinegar, which is available in Asian food stores and most large groceries.

Makes 1 cup

⅓ cup	miso paste	80 mL
¼ cup	mirin	60 mL
¼ cup	cider vinegar	60 mL
	juice of 1 lemon	
1 tbsp	freshly grated ginger	15 mL
2 tsp	minced garlic	10 mL
1 tsp	red chili flakes	5 mL

1. In a small bowl, combine all the ingredients with a whisk until well blended. This sauce will keep in the refrigerator for up to 2 weeks.

— *Moreka Jolar*

Hollyhock Oyster Barbecue Sauce

Bringing this thick barbecue sauce to a gentle simmer releases all the bold tastes and infuses it with hints of clove, cinnamon and allspice. This sauce is a taste sensation when spooned over an oyster on the half shell before grilling or baking. Also try marinating tofu or other seafood in it. The sauce will last a long time in the refrigerator and can be easily doubled to feed a crowd. If you like it hotter, add more hot chili sauce or cayenne.

Makes 1½ cups

¼ cup	tamari	60 mL
⅔ cup	tomato paste	160 mL
2 tbsp	lemon juice	30 mL
2 tbsp	molasses	30 mL
2 tbsp	brown sugar	30 mL
2 tbsp	cider vinegar	30 mL
1 tbsp	prepared Dijon mustard	15 mL
1 tbsp	Worcestershire sauce	15 mL
4-5	dashes of Tabasco sauce	4-5
1 tbsp	horseradish	15 mL
1	pinch each of cloves, cinnamon and allspice	1
	salt to taste	

1. Combine all the ingredients in a saucepan and bring them to a simmer, stirring constantly. Continue to simmer for about 10 minutes, allowing the flavors to combine. Cool and refrigerate.

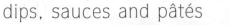

Mexican Red Sauce

This authentic red sauce is a must to have around if you love Mexican foods. Use it on top of enchiladas (page 73) or add it to burritos, Spanish rice, or scrambled eggs.

1. Use a food processor to blend the onions and garlic with all the herbs and spices. Pulse it until everything is coarsely ground. Transfer this to a large heavy saucepan and sauté it in the oil for 15 minutes. Add the chopped tomatoes and allow the mixture to simmer for at least an hour.

— *Moreka Jolar*

Makes 7 cups

2 cups	coarse chopped onions	480 mL
1 tbsp	crushed garlic	15 mL
1 tsp	salt	5 mL
1 tsp	black pepper	5 mL
1 tsp	chopped fresh oregano	5 mL
1 tsp	chopped fresh basil	5 mL
1 tsp	chopped fresh marjoram	5 mL
1 tsp	chopped fresh sage	5 mL
½ tsp	cinnamon	2.5 mL
½ tsp	cumin	2.5 mL
½ tsp	mustard powder	2.5 mL
½ tsp	ground celery seed	2.5 mL
¼ tsp	ground cloves	1.2 mL
¼ cup	sunflower or safflower oil	60 mL
6 cups	chopped fresh tomatoes	1.4 L

Nut Butter Sauce

Here is a rich, creamy sauce with the tang of lime and ginger that turns rice noodles and steamed vegetables into a simple yet elegant meal.

1. Combine all the ingredients well with a whisk or in a blender. This sauce keeps refrigerated for up to 3 weeks.

— *Rowan Brooks*

Makes 2 cups

1 cup	almond, hazelnut, peanut or cashew butter	240 mL
½ cup	coconut milk	120 mL
¼ cup	tamari	60 mL
2 tbsp	minced garlic	30 mL
2 tbsp	freshly grated ginger	30 mL
	juice of 1 lime	
½ tsp	red chili pepper flakes	2.5 mL

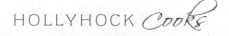

Roasted Red Pepper Sauce

Here are two easy ways to roast your own peppers. The sweet and smoky taste of this
elegant sauce will make it all worthwhile. Serve roasted red pepper sauce
over pasta, add some to your scrambled eggs, cook it with seafood,
or spread it on a sandwich.

Makes 3 cups

6	large red bell peppers	6
½	large eggplant	½
2 tbsp	crushed garlic	30 mL
1-2	seeded and diced jalapeños	1-2
	zest and juice of 1 lemon	
	salt and pepper to taste	

Preheat the oven to 350°F

1. Cut the eggplant in half lengthwise. Place 1 half only, open side down, onto an oiled baking sheet and bake until very soft through, approximately 1 hour. Allow it to cool.

2. Roast the peppers using one of the following two methods:

ROASTING PEPPERS ON A GAS BURNER

With gas or electric burners on high, place the whole peppers directly onto elements, 2 or 3 to each burner and allow them to roast over the heat. An overhead fan is essential for this fun activity. Use pair of metal tongs to turn the peppers and ensure that the peppers are roasted on each side until their skins have completely blackened and cracked and the flesh is soft. Transfer the roasted peppers to a bowl and cover it tightly with plastic wrap or a plastic bag. This allows the skins to peel off more easily. Allow the peppers to stand for 20 minutes under plastic before peeling the burnt skin off and removing the stalks and seeds.

ROASTING PEPPERS IN THE OVEN

Set the oven to broil. Place the whole peppers on a baking sheet under the broiler and bake them for about 20 minutes, turning the peppers until most of the skin has blackened. Transfer the peppers to a bowl while still hot and cover it tightly with plastic wrap or a plastic bag. Let the peppers sit for 20 minutes before peeling them and removing the stalks and seeds.

3. Spoon the baked eggplant meat out of its skin. In a food processor or blender, process the eggplant, roasted peppers and remaining ingredients until you reach a desired consistency. It's nice to leave some bits of pepper in for texture.

— Moreka Jolar

Sorrel Sauce for Salmon

Cooked sorrel possesses a lovely, lemony flavor which marries splendidly with salmon, but gets along well with other fish too, such as halibut, cod or snapper. This creamy sauce is worthy of a five-star rating.

1. Rinse the sorrel and remove the stems and center ribs. Chop finely.

2. In a large skillet, melt the butter on medium-low heat and sauté the chopped shallots or onion until softened, about 3-4 minutes. Add the chopped sorrel and continue to cook, stirring often until the sorrel is wilted and tender, about 5-10 minutes. Add the cream and bring to a simmer. Cook until it is slightly thickened. Season to taste with salt and pepper.

3. Spoon this warm sauce over cooked fish such as salmon or halibut and serve.

— *Hanyu Wasyliw*

Makes 1 cup

4 cups	fresh sorrel leaves	960 mL
1-2 tbsp	butter	15-30 mL
2	large, peeled and finely chopped shallots or ¼ cup minced onion	2
½ cup	heavy cream	120 mL
	salt and pepper to taste	

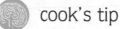 cook's tip

Be sure to use a non-reactive skillet such as stainless steel or a non-stick pan when cooking any greens. Aluminum or cast iron will discolor the greens.

Sweet Basil Tomato Sauce

Everyone loves a simple and classic tomato sauce teeming with fresh basil and chunky tomatoes. This sauce is versatile and can be served over pasta or rice, or cooked down and thickened to use as a pizza sauce.

1. In a large, heavy saucepan, sauté the onions, garlic, herbs and spices in the olive oil until they grow tender. Add the tomatoes and honey, cover and allow the mixture to simmer for at least an hour.

VARIATION
For a heartier sauce, add diced zucchini, carrots, celery, eggplant, mushrooms, chopped spinach or crumbled tofu.

— *Morcka Jolar*

Makes 7 cups

3 tbsp	olive oil	45 mL
2 cups	chopped onion	480 mL
1 tbsp	crushed garlic	15 mL
1 tsp	salt	5 mL
1 tsp	black pepper	5 mL
2 tsp	chopped fresh basil	10 mL
1 tsp	chopped fresh oregano	5 mL
6 cups	chopped fresh tomatoes	1.4 L
1 tbsp	honey	15 mL

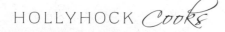

Thai Red Curry Sauce

Infusing the lime leaf in this classic curry sauce gives it its traditional Thai taste.
Lace it over Thai Peanut Tofu (page 75) for an aromatic meal.

Makes 2 cups

2 cups	coconut milk	480 mL
1 tsp	Thai red curry paste	5 mL
1	lime leaf *	1

1. In a heavy-bottomed saucepan, mix the red curry paste in to the coconut milk using a whisk. Add the lime leaf. Heat on low for approximately 30 minutes or until it starts to thicken slightly. Be careful not to allow the sauce to boil or it will separate. Use a heat diffuser. Add additional curry paste for more spice if you like.

* Lime leaves can be found dry or fresh frozen in most specialty food shops.

— *Moreka Jolar*

Caesar Tofu Dip or Salad Dressing

Our light, low-fat alternative to traditional Caesar dressing is firm enough to use as a dip for vegetables and bread sticks if chilled. Vegetarians will delight in the presence of the flavorings that stand in for anchovy, or one can add anchovies for the real thing.

Makes 1½ cups

1 cup	soft tofu	240 mL
2 tbsp	mayonnaise	30 mL
2 tbsp	yogurt	30 mL
1 tbsp	lemon juice	15 mL
2 tsp	Worcestershire sauce	10 mL
1 tsp	prepared Dijon mustard	5 mL
	dash of hot pepper sauce or cayenne	
¼ cup	grated Parmesan cheese	60 mL
1 tsp	crushed garlic	5 mL
1 tsp	olive oil	5 mL
	salt and pepper to taste	

1. In a food processor or blender, blend the tofu, mayonnaise, yogurt, lemon juice, Worcestershire sauce, Dijon mustard and hot pepper sauce until smooth. Transfer to a bowl and stir in the remaining ingredients. Chill before serving.

— *Debra Fontaine*

Fresh Curry Paste

This is a fresh and richly flavored alternative to commercial curry powders. Zing up your curry dish with a bit of this concentrated paste or use it as a condiment and spread a thin layer on a crisp cracker with a slice of Asiago cheese or garlic pickle. Whisk this fresh paste into coconut milk and marinate seafood in it or serve it over steamed vegetables and rice.

1. In a small saucepan, cover the yam generously with water and boil until tender. Drain and set aside.

2. In a small frying pan, sauté the ginger, garlic, salt, turmeric and cinnamon in a bit of oil for approximately 15 minutes. Set aside.

3. In a small, dry frying pan, gently toast all of the whole seeds until they begin to brown and smoke slightly. Allow them to cool for a while before finely grinding them in a coffee or spice grinder.

4. In a food processor, process the yams, sautéed mixture and all the ground spices into a thick paste. Store it in the fridge for up to 1 month or in a freezer for up to 6 months.

— *Rowan Brooks*

Makes 2 cups

2 cups	peeled and cubed yam	480 mL
½ cup	freshly grated ginger	120 mL
10	chopped cloves garlic	10
1 tsp	salt	5 mL
1 tsp	turmeric	5 mL
1 tsp	cinnamon	5 mL
2 tbsp	whole black mustard seeds	30 mL
2 tbsp	whole cumin seeds	30 mL
2 tbsp	whole coriander seeds	30 mL
1 tbsp	whole cardamom seeds	15 mL
2 tsp	whole fennel seeds	30 mL

 cook's tip

If you often grind whole spices and coffee beans, it may be to your advantage to have two separate grinders: one just for spices, seeds and nuts and one for coffee. This will ensure you don't have the rude awakening of cumin-spiced coffee in the morning!

Creamy Cheese Spreads

Here are some ideas for creating elegant spreads with soft chèvre or cream cheese.
These are easy and versatile and very impressive at the center of a cracker
plate. You can also spread them on bagels, in sandwiches, or toss them
with hot pasta for a rich pasta sauce.

Each recipe makes 2 ¾ cups of spread

CHÈVRE SPREAD

2 cups	chèvre *	240 mL

combined with any 1 of the following:

¾ cup	Roasted Red Pepper Sauce (page 104)	180 mL
¾ cup	of your favorite pesto (page 113)	180 mL
¾ cup	Green Olive Tapenade (page 109)	180 mL

SMOKED SALMON CREAM CHEESE SPREAD

2 cups	soft cream cheese	480 mL
1.75 oz.	flaked smoked salmon or lox	50 g
1 tbsp	chopped fresh dill	15 mL
2 tbsp	rinsed capers	30 mL

1. Use a fork or electric mixer to combine the cheese with the additions until the spread reaches a desired consistency. Chill and serve.

* Chèvre is soft goat's cheese.

— *Moreka Jolar*

Green Olive Tapenade

A tapenade is a classic French paste or spread made from black olives and, traditionally, capers and anchovies. This is a simplified and rustic version of that spread, with heaps of garlic and green olives instead of black ones. You can add a few chili flakes to turn up the heat. Serve this delicious spread on a French bread or focaccia (page 141), or as part of Roulade with Green Olive Tapenade (page 142). The tapenade keeps refrigerated for up to 2 weeks.

1. Process the ingredients in a food processor until they reach a desired consistency.

— *Moreka Jolar*

Makes 2 cups

2 cups	whole green olives	480 mL
1 tbsp	minced garlic	15 mL
½ cup	olive oil	120 mL

Hot Artichoke Dip

This rich and luxurious dip is topped with breadcrumbs and baked until bubbly and golden. Garnish it with a lemon wedge and serve it hot in the baking dish with crackers on the side.

Preheat the oven to 400°F.

1. In a small bowl, combine all the ingredients, except the breadcrumbs, and transfer the mixture to an ovenproof dish. Top with the breadcrumbs and bake until the dip bubbles and the top is brown.

— *Moreka Jolar*

Makes 3 cups

2 cups	finely chopped tinned or cooked artichoke hearts	480 mL
1 cup	finely grated Parmesan	240 mL
¾ cup	finely diced onions	180 mL
½ cup	yogurt	120 mL
½ cup	mayonnaise or Tofu Mayonnaise (page 119)	120 mL
1 tbsp	lemon juice	15 mL
½ tsp	black pepper	2.5 mL
¼ cup	breadcrumbs	60 mL

Hummus with Roasted Red Peppers

Chickpeas make this a protein-rich dip or spread. Here we combine roasted peppers
for a sweet edge and a pink tinge. With some Kalamata olives, sliced sundried tomatoes,
or a handful of fresh parsley, this hummus will provide a satisfying lunch.
Serve it with warm pita bread (page 140), vegetable sticks or
Middle Eastern Flatbread (page 135).

Serves 6-8

4 cups	cooked chickpeas	960 mL
¾ cup	fresh lemon juice	180 mL
½ cup	olive oil	120 mL
½ cup	toasted and ground sesame seeds	120 mL
I	roasted red bell pepper *	I
2 tbsp	crushed garlic	30 mL
	salt to taste	

1. Process the ingredients in a food processor or mash them with a potato masher until the hummus reaches a desired consistency.

* See (page 104) for instructions on how to roast peppers.

— *Moreka Jolar*

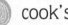 cook's tip

*Toasted and ground sesame seeds are a
great addition and condiment for all occasions. Toast the seeds in a dry frying pan
until brown, allow to cool, and grind in a
coffee grinder or food processor.*

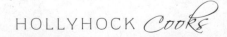

Lentil Spread with Walnuts and Curry

Protein-rich lentils serve as a base for this nutty, wholesome pâtè.
Serve will Middle Eastern Flatbread (page 135).

1. Combine all these ingredients in a food processor for about 10-15 seconds or mash all the ingredients with a potato masher. Chill and serve with crackers or spread it on a sandwich.

— *Moreka Jolar*

Makes 3 cups

2 cups	cooked brown lentils	480 mL
1 cup	whole toasted walnuts	240 mL
3 tbsp	olive oil	45 mL
3 tbsp	nutritional flake yeast	45 mL
1 tbsp	curry powder or Fresh Curry Paste (page 107)	15 mL 15 mL
2 tsp	crushed garlic	10 mL

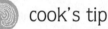 cook's tip

One cup of dry lentils will equal 2 cups of cooked. Rinse the lentils well and cover them generously with water and bring them to a boil. Reduce to simmer and cook until they are tender. Drain off the water.

Mushroom Miso Pâté

Vegetarian pâtès are always a treat. This thick and rich tasting spread has a hint of miso and the light crunch of toasted nuts and seeds. Garnish it with fresh parsley or oregano and serve it warm from the baking dish with bread or crackers on the side.

Makes 4 cups

4 cups	sliced mushrooms	960 mL
2 cups	chopped leeks or onions	480 mL
I cup	diced celery	240 mL
I tbsp	crushed garlic	15 mL
¼ cup	dry white wine	60 mL
I cup	whole toasted almonds	240 mL
I cup	toasted sunflower seeds	240 mL
¼ cup	water	60 mL
3 tbsp	miso paste	45 mL
2 tsp	black pepper	10 mL
I tsp	ground cumin	5 mL
I tsp	chopped fresh oregano	5 mL

Preheat the oven to 350°F.

1. In a large frying pan, sauté the mushrooms, leeks or onions, celery and garlic in wine until tender. Set aside.

2. Process the nuts and seeds in a food processor until they are coarsely chopped.

3. Add the sautéed vegetables and all the remaining ingredients to the nuts and seeds in the food processor and process until the mixture reaches a desired consistency. Press the pâté into a small ovenproof dish and bake for 20-30 minutes.

— *Moreka Jolar*

White Bean Spread with Roasted Garlic and Sage

This fine mixture of cannellini beans is a smooth and light spread with the bold taste of roasted garlic and a hint of sage. It is irresistible when served with Middle Eastern Flatbread (page 135) or spread onto any sandwich bread.

Makes 2 cups

4	cloves garlic	4
¼ cup	olive oil	60 mL
2 cups	cooked cannellini beans	480 mL
¼ cup	lemon juice	60 mL
I tsp	chopped fresh sage	5 mL
½ tsp	salt	2.5 mL

1. In a frying pan, roast the whole garlic cloves in the olive oil on medium heat until all the sides are dark brown.

2. In a food processor, place the cooked garlic cloves, the olive oil, the cooked beans and the remaining ingredients and process for approximately 10 to 15 seconds. Don't overdo the sage as it is very strong.

— *Moreka Jolar*

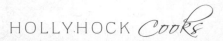

HOLLYHOCK *Cooks*

Cilantro Pesto with Sesame and Lime

In the tradition of pesto, this recipe combines the superb Asian ingredients of
cilantro, ginger, sesame and lime to make a bold and richly flavored,
versatile paste. Cilantro lovers will want to put this pesto on everything.
Toss it with hot soba noodles or rice, spread it on bruschetta and
sandwiches, or marinate seafood in it.

1. In a food processor, pulse the olive oil, cilantro, ginger, garlic and
jalapeño until well blended. Transfer to a bowl and stir in the sesame
seeds, lime juice and salt to taste and serve immediately.

VARIATION
Toasted and ground pine nuts or sunflower seeds can be used in place
of the sesame seeds.

* Extra virgin olive oil has a lighter flavor and is best used in fresh recipes
such as pesto and some dressings.

— *Moreka Jolar*

Makes 2 cups

¾ cup	extra virgin olive oil *	180 mL
1 cup	packed fresh cilantro	240 mL
2 tbsp	minced ginger	30 mL
1 tbsp	minced garlic	15 mL
½	seeded and minced jalapeño	½
¾ cup	toasted and ground sesame seeds	180 mL
	juice of 2 limes	
	salt to taste	

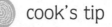 cook's tip

*The juice of a lemon and lime turns leafy
greens, such as basil, cilantro, steamed
spinach, and chard, brown. To avoid this,
be sure to add citrus juice just before
serving.*

Parsley and Pumpkin Seed Pesto

Toss this pesto with pasta or rice, spread it on a sandwich or bruschetta, or mix it with steamed vegetables. This versatile pesto is bright green and packed with the flavor of parsley and the nutty taste of the toasted pumpkin seeds. Pine nuts, almonds and sunflower seeds can stand in for the pumpkin seeds. Try adding Asiago cheese.

Makes 2 cups

2 cups	chopped fresh parsley, packed	480 mL
1 cup	extra virgin olive oil	240 mL
¼ cup	white wine vinegar or cider vinegar	60 mL
1½ cups	toasted pumpkin seeds	360 mL
2 tbsp	crushed garlic	30 mL
½ tsp	salt	2.5 mL

1. In a blender or food processor, pulse the parsley, olive oil and vinegar until coarsely chopped.

2. Add the toasted pumpkin seeds, garlic and salt and continue to pulse until the seeds are coarsely chopped. This pesto keeps refrigerated for up to 1 week.

— *Moreka Jolar*

 cook's tip

Pumpkin seeds are best toasted in a dry frying pan until they pop and turn brown. They are very rich in iron and are wonderful as a topping for salads and grains.

Sweet Basil Pesto with Toasted Almonds

At Hollyhock we get so excited in the kitchen when the mid-summer bounty of basil starts arriving from the garden. Fresh pesto begins showing up in all forms on the table. This pesto is wonderful on pasta and is equally delicious on steamed new potatoes or carrots. Spread it on bread as a treat in your sandwiches or bruschetta. Sautéeing the garlic brings out all its sugars and gives this pesto its distinctive sweet flavor.

1. In a small frying pan, gently sauté the garlic in ¼ cup of the olive oil until it is just turning brown. Set aside.

2. Put the remaining 1 cup of oil in a blender or food processor and pulse to mix in the basil leaves half a cup at a time. Be careful to just process until blended. Over-processing will bruise the basil and change the flavor of your pesto.

3. Transfer the basil mixture to a bowl and stir in the nuts and cheese. Serve immediately over hot pasta, rice or steamed new potatoes.

VARIATIONS
Pine nuts or sunflower seeds work well in place of almonds. Try other cheeses such as Romano or Asiago or no cheese at all. Add some chili flakes and lemon zest for zing. Add this pesto to flavor your tomato sauce.

— Moreka Jolar

Makes 2 cups

2 tbsp	coarsely chopped garlic	30 mL
1¼ cup	extra virgin olive oil	300 mL
1 cup	whole and packed fresh basil leaves	240 mL
¾ cup	toasted and finely chopped almonds	180 mL
1 cup	fresh finely grated Parmesan	240 mL

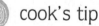 **cook's tip**

Pesto freezes beautifully. Pack the fresh pesto into containers or zip-lock bags, drizzle a bit of olive oil on top and seal well. This will keep frozen for up to 2 months.

Sundried Tomato Pesto

This pesto is vibrant and bold in taste and is delicious with pasta, rice, or spread in a sandwich. A thin layer on a baguette, sprinkled with some Asiago cheese and broiled makes an enticing bruschetta. If you like, add some creamy feta cheese and roasted vegetables, like peppers, asparagus, or onions to your pasta.

Makes 4 cups

4 oz.	sundried tomatoes or about 1 cup (240 mL) oil-packed	115 g
¼ cup	olive oil	60 mL
1 tbsp	grated lemon zest	15 mL
2 tsp	crushed garlic	10 mL
1 tsp	black pepper	5 mL
1 tsp	chili flakes	5 mL
¾ cup	water or water that the tomatoes have soaked in	180 mL
1½ cups	whole toasted walnuts	360 mL

1. If using dry tomatoes and not oil-packed, cover them with boiling water and allow them to stand for about 20 minutes, until tender. Reserve ¾ cup of this water when straining it off.

2. Put all the ingredients except for the nuts in a food processor or blender and process until it yields a thick paste. Add the nuts and process until it reaches a desired texture. Add more water to thin the pesto if you like.

— *Moreka Jolar*

Veggie Butter

The vibrant orange color and herb-filled taste set this butter apart from any other. Adding tomato paste and cooked carrots makes this a more nutritious, low-fat spread. To enrich its flavor, allow this butter to sit at room temperature for a few hours before serving. Serve with freshly baked bread.

Makes 2 cups

1½ cups	soft butter	360 mL
⅓ cup	tomato paste	80 mL
½ cup	cooked and mashed carrots	120 mL
¼ cup	finely chopped fresh chives	60 mL
3 tbsp	chopped fresh parsley	45 mL
2 tsp	chopped fresh basil	10 mL
2 tsp	chopped fresh oregano	10 mL
½ tsp	fresh thyme, if desired	2.5 mL

1. Blend all of the ingredients together with a mixer or fork until entirely mixed and soft.

VARIATION
Spice it up, if you like, with ½ tsp chili powder, 1 tsp lemon zest, or 1 tsp black pepper.

— *Moreka Jolar*

Herb Butter for Seafood

Garlic butter filled with flecks of fresh summer herbs is a great addition to all kinds of seafood. This butter can be used in a variety of ways. You can cook snapper, cod or halibut in it, or melt the butter and then dip prawns, clams or mussels in it.

1. Combine all the ingredients together with a fork. The butter keeps refrigerated for up to 2 weeks.

— *Jenica Rayne*

Makes ½ cup

½ cup	soft butter	120 mL
1 tbsp	chopped fresh basil	15 mL
1 tbsp	chopped fresh oregano	15 mL
1 tbsp	chopped fresh dill	15 mL
2 tsp	minced garlic	30 mL
½ tsp	black pepper	2.5 mL
	dash of cayenne pepper	

Sesame Dill Butter

Toasted sesame seeds combined with fresh dill create a magical fusion of tastes in this unique butter. Use it as a spread or cook seafood in it.

1. Mash the ingredients into the soft butter until everything is evenly combined.

— *Debra Fontaine*

Makes about ¼ cup

¼ cup	soft butter	60 mL
1 tsp	toasted sesame seeds	5 mL
2 tsp	chopped fresh dill	10 mL
1 tsp	chopped scallions	5 mL
1 tsp	soy sauce	5 mL
1 tsp	sesame oil	5 mL
	pinch of pepper	

Specialty Butters

Here are some ideas for adding a little extra pizzazz to simple butter. Savory, sweet, spicy and colorful — there's a butter for every occasion. Each recipe makes ½ cup or 120 mL.

Using ½ cup (120 mL) soft butter, blend in one of the following options:

HAZELNUT BUTTER

½ cup	toasted and ground hazelnuts	120 mL

Use on savory or sweet breads.

GARLIC-ROSEMARY BUTTER

2 tbsp	chopped fresh rosemary	30 mL
2 tsp	crushed garlic	30 mL

CHILI-LIME BUTTER

½ tsp	ancho chili powder	2.5 mL
1 tsp	lime zest	5 mL

This is excellent on corn on the cob.

PESTO BUTTER

3 tbsp	of your favorite pesto	45 mL
3 tbsp	grated Parmesan	15 mL

LEMON AND PEPPER BUTTER

1 tsp	lemon zest	5 mL
½ tsp	black pepper	2.5 mL

Try this with Savory Zucchini Muffins (page 144).

NASTURTIUM BUTTER

½ cup	chopped nasturtium petals	120 mL

This is wild and spicy on biscuits (page 125), like a party on your plate.

CHIVE-PUMPKIN SEED BUTTER

¼ cup	toasted and ground pumpkin seeds	60 mL
2 tbsp	chopped fresh chives	30 mL

BLOSSOM BUTTER

⅓ cup	chopped mixed edible flowers such as pansy, hollyhock, calendula, etc.	80 mL

HONEY-ROSE BUTTER

3 tbsp	honey	45 mL
⅓ cup	chopped fresh rose petals	80 mL

This is wonderful on Dreamy Whole Wheat Scones (page 128), muffins and pancakes.

— *Moreka Jolar*

Mayonnaise with Dijon and Tarragon

Homemade mayonnaise can be whipped up with astonishing ease and the flavor puts commercial mayonnaise to shame. Without additives and preservatives the taste is clean and fresh. This fresh mayonnaise will keep in the refrigerator for up to two weeks and can be laced with fresh tarragon or one of the other herb options.

1. In a blender or food processor, process the egg, vinegar, Dijon mustard, salt, pepper and tarragon for approximately 30 seconds, until blended. While mixing, drizzle in the oil in a steady stream. Stop mixing as soon as the oil has all been added.

— *Moreka Jolar*

Makes 1½ cups

1	egg	1
¼ cup	white wine vinegar	60 mL
2 tsp	prepared Dijon mustard	10 mL
½ tsp	salt	2.5 mL
½ tsp	black pepper	2.5 mL
¼ cup	either chopped fresh tarragon, garlic chives, parsley or oregano	60 mL
1 cup	sunflower or safflower oil	240 mL

Tofu Mayonnaise

This is an excellent, low-calorie and high-protein vegan alternative to traditional mayonnaise.

1. Combine all of the ingredients in a food processor or blender. Keep refrigerated.

— *Moreka Jolar*

Makes 2 cups

12 oz.	firm silken-style or regular soft tofu	340 g
⅓ cup	sunflower or safflower oil	80 mL
3 tbsp	tamari	45 mL
2 tbsp	lemon juice	30 mL
1 tsp	prepared Dijon mustard	5 mL
½ tsp	vegetable salts such as Spike or Herbamere	2.5 mL
¼ tsp	black pepper	1.2 mL

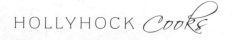

Raspberry Vinegar

This gourmet vinegar is easy to prepare, it just takes patience. Place a jar on the window ledge and allow the sweet raspberries to infuse the vinegar with their juice. The sweet fruit gives the vinegar a light, unique taste. Blackberries or loganberries will work as well and sugar is optional. These are the basic guidelines for making this vinegar. You can decide on the quantity to make.

raspberries

wine vinegar or rice vinegar

white sugar, if desired

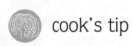 cook's tip

Vinegar is always best kept in a glass bottle with a cork or plastic lid as it will corrode and rust metal.

1. Fill a wide-mouth jar loosely with fresh, ripe raspberries and cover the fruit with a good quality wine vinegar or rice vinegar. Cover it with a lid and set it on a window ledge for 3-4 months. The sun helps the berries break down so they can infuse the vinegar with their sweet flavor.

2. When the vinegar is ready, use 3 layers of cheesecloth in a colander to strain off the remains of the fruit and reserve the liquid. Discard the berries.

VARIATIONS

If you would like a sweeter vinegar, follow these directions:

1. In a small saucepan, heat approximately one quarter of the flavored vinegar and add a half a cup of white sugar for every total of 5 cups of vinegar. Stir these until the sugar is dissolved. Add this to the rest of the vinegar and keep it in a cool place until ready for use.

— *Moreka Jolar*

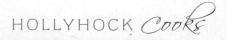

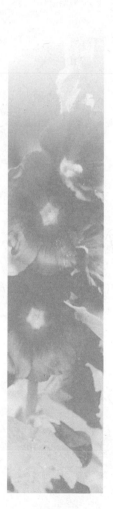

SIX

Baking

AT HOLLYHOCK, all of our baked goods are served fresh from the oven. The bread comes out onto the table steaming. Butter melts the instant it touches the surface of muffins or sweet breads and soaks into the warm grains of the buns. The smell of cakes and breads cooking in the oven wafts out of the kitchen and into the garden, enhancing bucolic summer days with enticing scents.

In the age of fast food, baking isn't something many of us take time for anymore. We turn to others to provide us with baking's pleasures and are happy if we live near stores that do it well. If we don't live near those stores, we turn to packaged, frozen baked goods that we reheat. We have little experience of what bread or pastry tastes like fresh out of any oven, much less our own, so we don't always know what we're missing.

We invite you to alter the course of North American evolution and experiment with an ancient and beautiful human art. Baking will take you back to the tastes that past generations knew and to flavors that pre-dated fast food, corporate farming, and multi-national grocery store chains. Just think what would happen to our society right now, if the hours per week the average North American spends watching TV were time spent baking. The transformation would be delicious.

Could baking become the meditation of the new century, with people of all ages visualizing world peace, human rights for all, more sustainable business practices, and solutions to environmental degradation, all with their baker's caps on?

With recipes like this, maybe so.

Babka with Cranberry-Almond Filling

Babka is a sweet, rich, yeasted bread from Poland. This babka is filled with a smooth almond paste and tart, dried cranberries, and then baked in an elegant spiral. It is a festive dish for any holiday.

Serves 8-10

DOUGH

½ cup	warm milk	120 mL
½ tsp	active dry yeast	2.5 mL
⅓ cup	white sugar	80 mL
½ cup	soft butter	20 mL
½ tsp	salt	2.5 mL
2	eggs	2
½ cup	sour cream	120 mL
1 cup	whole wheat flour	240 mL
3 cups	unbleached white flour	720 mL

FILLING

1 cup	dried cranberries, cherries, blueberries or currants	240 mL
2 cups	toasted and ground almonds	480 mL
¾ cup	melted butter	180 mL
½ cup	brown sugar	120 mL
1	egg	1
½ tsp	almond extract	2.5 mL
1 tsp	vanilla extract	5 mL

 cook's tip

To achieve that special shine on your baked goods, simply brush the top with milk or equal portions milk and whipped egg just before baking.

DOUGH

1. You can prepare the dough early in the day or the day before. Using a medium-sized bowl, dissolve just 1 tbsp of the white sugar in the milk and sprinkle the yeast over this. Allow it to stand until foamy, about 15 minutes.

2. In a larger bowl, beat the butter and the remaining sugar with a fork. Add the salt, eggs, sour cream and the yeast sponge and continue to mix well. Use a wooden spoon to stir in the whole wheat flour and begin to add the white flour. Stir until you can work the dough with your hands and then transfer it to a lightly floured surface and gently knead in the remaining flour. This dough will remain sticky. Shape the dough into a ball and place it in a lightly buttered bowl, cover with a damp towel and allow it to rise about 2 hours, or until the dough is doubled its original size. At this point the dough can also be refrigerated overnight.

FILLING

3. To make the filling, place the dried berries in a small bowl and cover them with boiling water. Soak them until they're soft, for about 20 minutes, then drain off the water. Set aside. In another bowl, combine the remaining filling ingredients; mix thoroughly.

ASSEMBLY

4. On a lightly floured surface, use a rolling pin to roll out the dough into a rectangle approximately ¼-inch thick. If your dough has been refrigerated, allow it to warm up for 20 minutes before attempting to roll it out. Spread the nut filling evenly over the dough and sprinkle the dried berries over this. Roll the dough up as if you were rolling up cinnamon buns and pinch the dough at the seam. On a lightly buttered baking sheet or parchment paper, shape this snake-like roll into a loose spiral and score or slash the top in a few places with a sharp knife. Cover it with a damp cloth and allow it to rise another 1 hour in a warm spot.

5. Preheat the oven to 350°F. Use a pastry brush to brush the entire loaf with a milk or egg wash. Bake for 1 hour or until golden on the top and sides. Allow it to cool slightly on a cooling rack before cutting and serving.

— *Moreka Jolar*

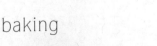
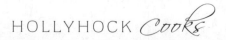 HOLLYHOCK *Cooks*

Basic Whole Wheat Pastry

There is nothing quite like a perfect rich and flaky pastry. Here is the ideal recipe and now the rest is in your hands. The key to successful pastry is to handle it as little as possible. The double crust recipe will yield enough pastry for the top and bottom crust of a fruit pie such as Apple Berry Pie (page 151). The single crust recipe yields enough pastry for a bottom crust and can be used in such recipes as Shrimp and Braised Leek Tart (page 68), Mediterranean Garlic Custard Tart (page 60) or your favorite quiche.
Both recipes are for a 9-inch pie plate.

DOUBLE CRUST

1. In a medium-sized bowl, combine all the dry ingredients well. Use a pastry cutter or 2 knives to cut in the butter. Work this mixture until it is crumbly and in pea-sized bits. Avoid handling it with your hands or the fragile pastry will turn doughy.

2. In a measuring cup, beat the egg with the vinegar and add enough cold water to this to equal a half a cup of liquid. Pour this over the flour mixture and toss gently with your hands. Do not knead. Mix only until you can form the pastry into a firm ball. The key to good pastry is to handle it as little as possible. Wrap the ball completely in plastic wrap or wax paper and chill it for 1 hour before rolling it out with a rolling pin.

SINGLE CRUST

1. Follow the same instructions for the double crust. This recipes does not include the egg or vinegar as it would be just too much liquid. Omit the sugar if you are using this pastry for a savory quiche or tart.

— *Moreka Jolar*

DOUBLE CRUST

1 cup	whole wheat pastry flour	240 mL
¾ cup	unbleached white flour	180 mL
2 tbsp	white sugar	30 mL
1 tsp	salt	5 mL
1 cup	soft butter or vegetable shortening	240 mL
1	egg	1
1 tbsp	white vinegar	15 mL

SINGLE CRUST

½ cup	whole wheat pastry flour	120 mL
⅔ cup	unbleached white flour	160 mL
1 tbsp	white sugar	15 mL
¼ tsp	salt	1.2 mL
½ cup	soft butter or vegetable shortening	120 mL
2 tbsp	cold water	30 mL

 cook's tip

If wrapped tightly in plastic, this pastry dough will keep frozen for up to a month. Allow several hours to thaw before rolling it out.

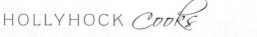 

Best Ever Cornbread

This golden cornbread is flecked with green jalapeños and red bell peppers.
It is a moist, rich and quick dinner bread that is the perfect
accompaniment to soup, stew or a Mexican meal.

Serves 12-15

2 cups	finely diced onions	480 mL
I cup	finely diced red bell peppers	240 mL
2 cups	fresh or frozen corn	480 mL
I	seeded and minced jalapeño	I
I tsp	black pepper	5 mL
I cup	chopped fresh parsley	240 mL
I cup	soft butter	240 mL
½ cup	brown sugar	120 mL
5	eggs	5
I cup	shredded Monterey Jack cheese	240 mL
½ cup	whole wheat flour	120 mL
½ cup	unbleached white flour	120 mL
I cup	yellow cornmeal	240 mL
I ½ tbsp	baking powder	17.5 mL
¼ tsp	salt	1.2 mL

1. In a large frying pan, sauté the onions, bell peppers, corn, jalapeño, black pepper and parsley until everything is very tender. Set aside.

2. Preheat the oven to 350°F. In a large bowl, cream the butter and brown sugar together. Whisk in the eggs and cheese.

3. In a separate bowl, combine all the dry ingredients together. Gently add the dry mixture to the wet and fold in with a wooden spoon. Mix in the sautéed vegetables to the batter. Spread this thick batter evenly into a lightly oiled 9x13-inch baking dish. Bake for 30-35 minutes, until a knife comes out of the center clean. Allow the cornbread to cool completely before cutting.

VARIATIONS
Alternative flours such as spelt can be used in place of the whole wheat and white flours, and the cheese can be omitted.

— *Moreka Jolar*

" *The food at Hollyhock is tasty,
cooked with care and love. I
take away a soft sweetness and
a fat stomach!"*
— *Ram Dass*

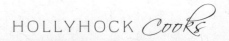

Buttermilk Herb Biscuits

These flaky, savory biscuits served warm will make any meal a special occasion. If you like, add a half a cup of shredded sharp cheddar or other cheese or a handful of bright orange or yellow calendula flower petals with the herbs.

Preheat the oven to 350°F.

1. In a large bowl, mix all the dry ingredients together.

2. Use a pastry cutter or 2 knives to cut in the butter to the dry ingredients until the mix is in pea-sized shapes. Add the parsley and scallions.

3. Pour in the buttermilk and toss the mixture gently with your hands, just until it starts to stick together. Do not over-mix.

4. Shape the dough into a ball, but do not knead, and use a rolling pin to roll it out on a lightly floured surface until it is a ½-inch thick. Cut with a round cookie cutter or a drinking glass. Place each biscuit on a lightly oiled baking sheet or parchment paper. Bake just until they start to brown, for about 15-20 minutes.

— *Debra Fontaine*

Makes 8

½ cup	whole wheat flour	120 mL
½ cup	white flour	120 mL
1 tsp	baking powder	5 mL
1 tsp	sugar	5 mL
¼ tsp	salt	1.2 mL
¼ tsp	baking soda	1.2 mL
2½ tbsp	butter	32.5 mL
¼ cup	chopped fresh parsley	60 mL
¼ cup	diced scallions	60 mL
½ cup	buttermilk	120 mL

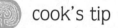 **cook's tip**

In a pinch without a rolling pin? Simply fill a clean wine bottle with ice water, cork it and use it to roll out any dough or pastry.

Caraway Rye Bread

This quick bread is easy and fast to prepare and the end result is a dark, moist loaf encrusted with whole oats. Tofu Salad (page 26) is an excellent spread for this wholesome bread.

Serves 10-12

3 cups	whole wheat flour	720 mL
I cup	rye flour	240 mL
2 tsp	whole caraway seeds	10 mL
2 tsp	baking soda	10 mL
I tsp	baking powder	5 mL
I tsp	salt	5 mL
2 tbsp	vinegar	30 mL
1½ cups	milk or dairy alternative	360 mL
I	egg beaten	I
2 tbsp	molasses	30 mL
	a handful of oats	

Preheat the oven to 375°F.

1. In a large bowl, combine all the dry ingredients.

2. In a large measuring cup, mix the vinegar with the milk. This will make it sour and curdle slightly. Whisk in the egg and molasses to the sour milk mixture. Use a large wooden spoon to completely stir the wet mixture into the dry mixture. The dough will remain very sticky.

3. Place a handful of oats on a dry surface. With floured hands, shape the dough into a vague loaf shape and roll it in the oats before placing it in a lightly oiled loaf pan. Bake for about an hour, or until a toothpick comes out of the center clean.

— *Moreka Jolar*

cook's tip

Slice breads and bagels before freezing and freeze them in air-tight bags. To minimize freezer burn, use a straw to suck all the air out before zipping the bag closed. When the bread or bagels are removed from the freezer, they're easy to separate into slices and pop into the toaster to thaw.

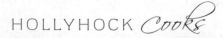

Crispy Cheese Crackers

These versatile crackers are a favorite with all ages yet elegant enough to serve at a
cocktail party. To vary the recipe, after chilling the dough, roll the log in
poppyseeds or cracked black pepper to give each cracker a classy edge,
or shape the log into a long heart and slice it for individual
heart-shaped crackers.

1. In a small bowl, use a fork to combine the grated cheese with the soft
   butter. Add the mustard and flour and work well with your hands until
   you can shape the dough into a firm log, approximately 1½ inches in
   diameter. Wrap the log tightly in wax paper or plastic wrap, seal the
   ends and refrigerate for at least 2 hours.

2. Preheat the oven to 375°F. Unwrap the log of dough and use a sharp
   knife to slice it into ¼-inch thin rounds. Lay these on a baking sheet and
   bake until they are bubbly and brown, approximately 10-15 minutes.
   Cool completely on a cooling rack.

   — Moreka Jolar

Makes about 2 dozen

4 oz.	finely grated Sardo, Swiss, Parmesan, sharp cheddar or other cheese	115 g
4 tbsp	soft butter	60 mL
1 tsp	mustard powder	5 mL
½ cup	unbleached white flour	120 mL

*" Hollyhock is feeding healthy,
sustainable and diverse food
to the social movements that
are working to build a new
culture that reflects those very
values. Hollyhock is feeding the
movement for a better world. "*
— Karen Mahon

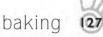

Dreamy Whole Wheat Scones

These whole wheat scones are nutritious and hearty, while retaining a light, flaky texture. The trick to making a good flaky scone is not to over-mix. This batter likes to go immediately into the oven. This is a very forgiving and versatile recipe and nine flavor variations are given here. After you've tried this recipe a few times and you are more confident, try using yogurt or milk as a lighter alternative to buttermilk or cream. These quantities will vary.

Makes approximately 10

3 cups	whole wheat flour or spelt	720 mL
⅓ cup	sugar	80 mL
2½ tsp	baking powder	12.5 mL
1 tsp	baking soda	5 mL
¾ cup	butter or margarine	180 mL
1¾ cups	buttermilk, cream, or dairy alternative	420 mL

1½ cups (360 mL) of 1 of these options

• blueberries with 1 tbsp (15 mL) orange zest

• thinly sliced candied ginger

• raspberries with 1 tbsp (15 mL) lemon zest

• grated sharp cheddar cheese and 1 tbsp (15 mL) black pepper

• a mix of sesame, sunflower and pumpkin seeds

• chopped fresh cranberries

• dried currants or apricots with 2 tsp (10 mL) star anise

• chopped dried dates with 1 tbsp (15 mL) orange zest

• chopped roasted walnuts with a maple syrup glaze

Preheat the oven to 425°F.

1. In a large bowl, mix the flour, sugar, baking powder and baking soda. Using a pastry cutter or knife, cut in the butter until the mixture is crumbly and pea sized. Mix in the berries, nuts or your choice of optional ingredients.

2. Pour all the buttermilk over this mixture and gently toss about with your hands. (Hands really are the best tool for this.) Do not over-mix. There should still be lumps of flour in the batter.

3. Use a spoon or ice cream scoop to divide the batter into roughly 10 scones on a lightly oiled baking sheet or parchment. Bake for 12-15 minutes, until golden and firm to the touch. Allow the scones to cool for 5 minutes before transferring them to cooling rack.

— *Moreka Jolar*

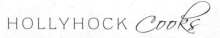

Fennel-Topped French Bread

This is a classic, chewy, white French bread topped with aromatic fennel seeds.
These loaves take a bit of work to prepare, but the final result is well worth the effort.
The bread freezes well, so cook a few batches and put a couple away.

1. In a large bowl, dissolve the sugar in the warm water. Add 2 cups of the flour and the yeast. Whisk or beat with a wooden spoon, until the flour and yeast are well combined with the water. Cover with a clean tea towel and leave it to proof for about 20 minutes in a warm spot.

2. The sponge will now be active and bubbly. Stir it down with a wooden spoon and add the tablespoon of salt. Beat in another couple of cups of flour, until you can handle the dough. Transfer it to a dry surface and knead in the remaining flour until you have smooth, elastic dough. Place the dough in a large, lightly oiled bowl, cover it with a damp towel and let it rise in a warm spot for about 1 hour, or until the dough has doubled in bulk.

3. Preheat the oven to 450°F. Sprinkle a large cookie sheet with cornmeal. Punch down the dough to release the air bubbles and knead it for a minute or so. Use a sharp knife to divide the dough into 2 equal pieces. Pat down 1 piece of dough or use a rolling pin to shape the dough into a rough rectangle. Roll it up like a jellyroll, pinch the bottom seam and place it seam-side down on the baking sheet. Repeat with the second loaf. Both loaves will fit on 1 cookie sheet. Cover them with a tea towel and let them rise in a warm spot until approximately doubled in size. This will only take 10-12 minutes.

4. Use a sharp knife or exacto blade to make 4 or 5 diagonal slashes on the top of each loaf and then brush the tops with the egg-white mixture. Sprinkle them with fennel seeds and coarse salt. Place them in the hot oven.

5. After 10 minutes, spray the bread with a spritz of water from a clean plant sprayer. Do this a couple more times while the bread is baking to create the steam that gives the bread its chewy, crisp crust. Bake for 30 to 40 minutes until the bread is golden and sounds hollow when the bottom is tapped. Cool on a rack.

— *Hanyu Wasyliw*

Makes 2 French loaves

2½ cups	warm water	600 mL
1 tbsp	sugar	15 mL
2 tbsp	rapid-rise yeast	30 mL
5½-6 cups	unbleached flour	1.3-1.4 L
1 tbsp	salt	15 mL
	cornmeal for the baking sheet	
1	egg white, beaten with 1 tbsp water	1
1-2 tbsp	whole fennel seeds	15-30 mL
1 tbsp	coarse sea salt or kosher salt	15 mL

 cook's tip

Place a pan with about 1 inch of hot water on the bottom rack of the oven. A square or rectangular cake pan works well. This creates steam, which will give a crisp and chewy crust to your yeasted breads.

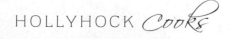

Granary Buns

These charming, round buns are nutritious and hearty with a bold rye flavor. They are
the perfect partner for Lemon-Lentil Soup (page 46) or Borscht (page 35).

Makes 12-16 buns

I cup	milk	240 mL
½ cup	packed brown sugar	120 mL
2 tbsp	butter	30 mL
2 tsp	salt	10 mL
I cup	warm water	240 mL
I tsp	sugar	5 mL
I tbsp	active dry yeast	15 mL
2 cups	whole wheat flour	480 mL
I cup	rye flour	240 mL
2 cups	unbleached white flour	480 mL
I	egg yolk	I
2 tbsp	water	30 mL
	a handful of rye or oat flakes	

1. In a small saucepan, heat the milk, brown sugar, butter and salt until the butter melts. Allow it to cool until it is lukewarm.

2. In a large bowl, dissolve the teaspoon of sugar in the warm water. Add the yeast and proof for 10 minutes until foaming.

3. Add the milk mixture to the yeast mixture. Use a wooden spoon to stir in the whole wheat flour and rye flour. Continue to add white flour until the dough is stiff enough to handle and then transfer it to a dry surface and knead in the remaining flour. Knead for approximately 10 minutes until the dough is smooth and elastic. Add additional white flour, if necessary, to make a stiff dough. Place the dough in a lightly oiled bowl and cover it with a damp towel. Let it rise in a warm spot until doubled in size, about 1½ hours.

4. Punch the dough down and knead it for a couple of minutes. Cut the dough into 12 to 16 equal pieces and form it into balls. Place the balls 2 inches apart on a lightly oiled baking sheet. Cover with the damp towel and let them rise in a warm spot for another hour.

5. Preheat the oven to 350°F. In a small bowl, whisk together the egg yolk and 2 tbsp of water. Brush the egg wash on to the buns and sprinkle them with rye or oat flakes, or both. Bake for 20 minutes. Cool on a cooling rack.

— *Carmen Rosse*

HOLLYHOCK *Cooks*

Hollyhock Bread

This nutritious bread has become a tradition since Hollyhock's conception.
Now guests who visit the toast bar consume 20 to 30 loaves of this hearty bread each week.
Packed with grains and seeds, and with a bold, nutty flavor,
Hollyhock Bread makes excellent toast, sandwiches, croutons and breadcrumbs.
Each slice is perfect for slathering with nut butter, honey and
local fruit preserves.

1. In a large bowl, dissolve the honey and molasses in the warm water. Sprinkle the yeast over this and let it stand for 15 minutes until foamy. Add the millet, oats, bran, seeds, salt and white flour and stir well with a wooden spoon. Slowly stir in whole wheat flour, 1 cup a time.

2. When the dough is firm enough to handle, turn it onto a dry surface and knead in the flour until you can punch your dry fist in and bring it out clean. You will knead for about 10 minutes. Transfer the dough to a lightly floured or oiled bowl and cover with a damp towel. Allow it to rise in a warm spot until it has doubled in size, approximately 1 hour.

3. Turn the dough onto a lightly floured surface and knead out all the air pockets for about 2 minutes. Divide the dough into 2 equal portions, shape into loaves and place into lightly oiled loaf pans. Use a sharp knife to score the tops of the loaves with 3 or 4 diagonal slashes. Re-cover with the damp towel and let them rise another 45 minutes.

4. Preheat the oven to 350°F. Bake the loaves for approximately 1 hour until they are very brown on top. Turn the bread out of the loaf pans and allow them to cool on a cooling rack.

Makes 2 loaves

2 cups	warm water	480 mL
1 tbsp	honey	15 mL
1 tbsp	molasses	15 mL
2 tsp	yeast	10 mL
½ cup	millet	120 mL
½ cup	oats	120 mL
¼ cup	wheat bran or bran flakes	60 mL
¼ cup	sunflower seeds	60 mL
¼ cup	sesame seeds	60 mL
¼ cup	flax seeds	60 mL
1 tsp	salt	5 mL
1½ cups	white flour	360 mL
3 cups	whole wheat flour	720 mL

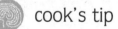 cook's tip

To test the readiness of most breads, pull the bread out of the pan and tap the side and bottom of the loaf with a wooden spoon or your knuckles. Bread that is ready will sound hollow. You can also pierce the bread with a cooking thermometer to test its readiness. Bread will have an interior temperature of 200°F when it is done.

 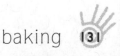

Honey Curry Bread

This is a rich, moist, savory bread with a sweet honey tone and a golden curry color. The braided loaf is a perfect companion to Carrot Soup with Tahini (page 37) or Spicy Squash Soup with Roasted Garlic and Yogurt (page 43).

Makes 1 loaf

¼ cup	warm water	60 mL
1½ tbsp	yeast	23 mL
⅓ cup	honey	80 mL
2 tbsp	butter	30 mL
1 tsp	salt	5 mL
1 tbsp	curry powder	15 mL
1 cup	buttermilk	240 mL
1 cup	whole wheat flour	240 mL
3½ cups	white flour	840 mL
1	egg	1
	a handful of slivered almonds	

> " *Breaking bread together is an ancient act that confirms all of us in our essential humanity. We are sharing even if we don't know each other or speak.* "
> — *Sharon Butala*

1. In a large bowl, dissolve just 1 tbsp of the honey in warm water and sprinkle the yeast over this. Allow it to sit for 10 minutes until foamy.

2. Meanwhile, in a small saucepan, melt the butter with the remaining honey, salt and curry powder. Add the melted butter mixture and the buttermilk to the yeast sponge and use a wooden spoon to stir in the whole wheat flour. Continue to add the white flour. When the dough is stiff enough to handle, transfer it to a lightly floured surface and continue to knead in the remaining flour until the dough is firm but remains sticky. Shape the dough into a ball and place it in a lightly oiled bowl. Cover it with a damp towel and allow it to rise in a warm place until it has doubled in size, about 1 hour.

3. Punch down the dough, shape it into a loaf or divide it into 3 equal pieces and braid it and put it in a lightly oiled loaf pan. Cover it with a damp towel again and allow it to rise for another 45 minutes.

4. Preheat the oven to 375°F. Whip the egg and brush the loaf lightly with the beaten egg. Sprinkle with slivered almonds. Bake for 40-45 minutes, until golden brown on top. Allow the bread to cool in the loaf pan for 10 minutes before inverting it onto a cooling rack.

— *Rosemary Wooldridge*

Honey Wheat Bagels

A bagel just isn't a bagel if it's not boiled! It needs no oil or egg or milk just a quick stovetop bath to achieve the chewy skin and soft insides that separate bagels from any other bread. Serve fresh bagels with a cream cheese or chèvre variation, Green Olive Tapenade (page 109) or Blossom Butter (page 118).

1. In a large bowl, dissolve the honey in the water, sprinkle the yeast over this and allow it to stand until the yeast has dissolved and is foamy, approximately 15 minutes.

2. In a small bowl, combine the salt with the white flour and stir into the yeast sponge. Begin to add whole wheat flour, 1 cup at a time, stirring well with a wooden spoon. When the dough is firm enough to handle, transfer it to a lightly floured surface and knead for 10 minutes. Form the dough into a ball, place it in a lightly oiled large bowl, cover it with a damp towel or plastic wrap and set it in a warm spot to rise for approximately 1½ hours or until the dough is twice its original volume.

3. When the dough has finished rising, start to prepare to boil your bagels. Preheat the oven to 425°F. Fill a large pot with water and bring it to a rolling boil. A wok works really well for this. Have ready another pot full with cold water and 1 tray of ice cubes. Also have your toppings of choice spread in a low dish for dipping each bagel in. Have ready a couple of un-oiled baking sheets.

4. Punch down your dough and knead it a few times before dividing it into 12 equal portions. Using the palms of your hands, roll each piece into "snakes" that will wrap around the width of your hand. Use a bit of flour if it's sticky. Pinch the ends really firmly together and rest the bagel on a well-oiled cutting board while you shape the other bagels.

5. Place the bagels, 3 at a time, into the boiling water. If necessary, cover the pot to keep a rolling boil. Boil for 3 minutes, turning a few times. Use a slotted spoon to remove the bagels and place in the ice bath for 30 seconds.

6. Allow each bagel to drip a bit before dipping the top into your favorite topping and place the bagels on the cookie sheet, seeds or topping facing up, and with 2 inches of space between each bagel. Continue with this process until you've filled a baking sheet. Bake for approximately 40 minutes, until well browned. Cool the bagels on a cooling rack or eat them warm.

— *Moreka Jolar*

Makes 1 dozen

2½ cups	warm water	600 mL
⅓ cup	honey	80 mL
2 tsp	active dry yeast	10 mL
1½ cups	unbleached white flour	360 mL
2 tsp	salt	10 mL
5½ cups	whole wheat flour	1.3 L
1 tray	ice cubes, for chilling	1 tray

TOPPING VARIATIONS

hulled sesame seeds

poppyseeds

dry onion flakes

dry minced garlic flakes

Use one of the above or combine them all.

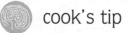 cook's tip

If your bagels wrinkle after baking, they've been boiled for too long. If the hole closes and pops up during baking, they've not been boiled long enough. Be patient and you'll get the feel for it.

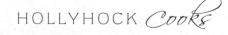

Lemon Blueberry Muffins

These blueberry muffins can be a delicious start to your day or a wonderful pick-me-up with afternoon tea. Add a cup of pineapple chunks for more moistness and sweetness.

Makes 1 dozen

1½ cups	whole wheat flour	360 mL
1 cup	white flour	240 mL
⅔ cup	brown sugar	160 mL
2 tsp	baking powder	10 mL
1 tsp	baking soda	5 mL
2 tbsp	lemon or orange zest	30 mL
½ cup	soft butter	120 mL
2 cups	fresh or partially thawed blueberries	480 mL
2 cups	yogurt	480 mL
2	eggs	2
½ cup	shredded coconut	120 mL

Preheat the oven to 400°F.

1. In a large bowl, combine all the dry ingredients. Use a pastry cutter or 2 knives to cut in the butter. Add the blueberries and, if you wish, a cup of pineapple chunks.

2. In a small bowl, whisk together the yogurt and eggs. Use a wooden spoon to gently fold the wet mixture into the dry. Be careful not to over-mix. The batter should remain a bit lumpy.

3. Divide the batter into 12 portions in lightly oiled muffin tins or use muffin papers to line the tins. Sprinkle the tops with the coconut. Bake for 20-25 minutes until golden and firm to the touch. Allow the muffins to cool for a few minutes before lifting them out of the tins.

— *Linda Gardner*

 cook's tip

Don't let your breads and muffins sweat. As soon as you can lift fresh breads and muffins off of baking sheets and out of loaf pans, transfer them to a cooling rack to avoid a moist condensation that will turn your fresh breads soggy.

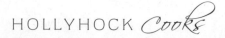

Middle Eastern Flatbread
with Cumin Seeds

This is a crisp whole-wheat cracker that is excellent with Hummus (page 110) or White Bean Dip (page 112). The whole wheat yeasted dough is rolled out very thinly and baked fast to create a nice crisp cracker. Use sesame seeds in place of cumin seeds for a more versatile recipe.

1. In a medium-sized bowl, dissolve the sugar in the warm water and sprinkle the yeast over it. Allow it to foam for 15 minutes.

2. Add the cold water, salt, cumin seeds and 1 cup of the whole wheat flour. Stir well with a wooden spoon. Continue to stir in another cup of whole wheat flour until the dough is stiff enough so that you can transfer it to a clean surface and knead in the remaining flour. Knead for 5 minutes and form the dough into a ball and place it in a lightly oiled bowl. Cover it with a damp cloth and place it in a warm spot to rise for 1 hour or until the dough doubles in size.

3. Preheat the oven to 350°F. Punch down the dough and cut it into 4 equal pieces. Knead 1 piece a few times before rolling it out with a rolling pin on a well-floured surface to form a thin, approximately 9x12-inch, rectangle. Place it on a lightly oiled cookie sheet. Continue this with remaining 3 balls of dough. You may be able to fit 2 per baking sheet.

4. Bake at 350°F for approximately 20 minutes, until the crackers begin to grow crisp and brown. Cool the flatbreads on a cooling rack before breaking them into generous-sized crackers.

— *Chloe Gregg*

Serves 10-15

½ cup	warm water	120 mL
1 tsp	brown sugar	5 mL
1 tsp	active dry yeast	5 mL
½ cup	cold water	120 mL
1 tsp	salt	5 mL
2 tsp	whole cumin seeds	10 mL
2⅓ cups	whole wheat flour	560 mL

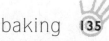

Mom's Rhubarb Coffee Cake

The Hollyhock garden yields bucketfuls of rhubarb in the spring. What better way to eat up this glorious tart stalk than in a scrumptious coffee cake? Serve it warm topped with Applesauce Tahini Pudding (page 176).

Serves 15-20

I cup	brown sugar	240 mL
½ cup	soft butter or shortening	120 mL
I	egg	I
I tsp	vanilla extract	5 mL
2 cups	fresh rhubarb cut in 1-inch pieces	480 mL
2 cups	unbleached white flour	480 mL
I tsp	baking soda	5 mL
I tsp	cinnamon	5 mL
½ tsp	salt	2.5 mL
I cup	milk, buttermilk or soymilk	240 mL

TOPPING

¼ cup	soft butter	60 mL
½ cup	brown sugar	120 mL
½ cup	shredded coconut	120 mL

Preheat the oven to 350°F.

1. In a large bowl, cream the butter and the sugar together. Add the egg and vanilla and mix well.

2. In another bowl, combine ½ cup of the flour with the rhubarb and mix to coat the fruit with flour. Set aside.

3. In a separate medium-sized bowl, combine the remaining flour and other dry ingredients. Mix well.

4. In a small bowl, mix the topping ingredients with a fork or pastry cutter. Set aside.

5. Add the dry ingredients, alternating with the milk, to the egg mixture. Mix just until combined. Fold the rhubarb into the batter and pour into a lightly oiled 9x13-inch baking pan. Sprinkle the topping over this and bake for 45 minutes or until a wooden skewer comes out of the center clean. Allow to cool slightly before cutting.

— *Ted Wallbridge*

cook's tip

Here is an old cost-effective tip. Keep the wrappers from your butter in the freezer and whip one out to rub onto and lightly butter a baking dish before use, instead of investing in costly, environmentally unfriendly aerosol cans.

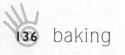
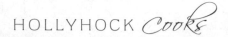

Oatmeal Muffins

This muffin recipe is excellent because it is so versatile and forgiving. The fun is in the filling. Take your pick of the eight variations suggested below or invent your own combination. These muffins are great at breakfast or any time of day. For a non-dairy muffin, replace the buttermilk with a non-dairy milk or yogurt, juice or even water. Serve with Honey Rose Butter (page 118).

Preheat the oven to 400°F.

1. In a large bowl, combine the oats and buttermilk and let them sit for 10 minutes. Gradually add the oil, brown sugar and the egg, one ingredient at a time, stirring each one in well with a wooden spoon.

2. In a separate bowl, combine the flour, salt, baking soda and baking powder. Gently stir the dry ingredients into the wet and now add your favorite flavor combination. Do not over-mix; there should still be some lumps in the batter.

3. Scoop the batter into a lightly oiled muffin tin or muffin papers and bake for 20-25 minutes or until firm to the touch. Allow the muffins to cool for 5 minutes before lifting them out of the tin.

FILLING VARIATIONS
1 cup (240 mL) of 1 of these options:

- thinly sliced apple with 1 tsp (5 mL) each of cinnamon and nutmeg
- chopped dates with 1 tsp (5 mL) orange zest and a pinch of cloves
- diced banana with 1 tsp (5 mL) mace
- grated cheese
- chopped pear with 2 tsp (10 mL) fresh grated ginger
- diced mango with ½ cup (60 mL) shredded coconut
- diced banana with ¾ cup (180 mL) chocolate chips
- a mix of toasted pumpkin, sesame, sunflower and poppyseeds

— *Dianne West*

Makes 1 dozen

1 cup	rolled oats	240 mL
1 cup	buttermilk	240 mL
½ cup	sunflower or safflower oil	120 mL
½ cup	brown sugar	120 mL
1	egg beaten	1
1 cup	unbleached white flour	240 mL
1 tsp	salt	5 mL
½ tsp	baking soda	2.5 mL
1 tsp	baking powder	5 mL

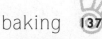

Pear Coffee Cake

The crunchy streusel topping on the sweet pear halves will make a tremendous breakfast and a perfect match for a cup of freshly brewed organic coffee.

Serves 10-15

1 cup	soft butter	240 mL
1 cup	brown sugar	240 mL
4	eggs	4
1½ tbsp	lemon zest	23 mL
1¾ cups	unbleached white flour	420 mL
2 tsp	baking powder	10 mL
56 fl. oz.	pear halves in juice	1.6 L

STREUSEL

½ cup	flour	120 mL
½ cup	soft butter	120 mL
1 cup	brown sugar	240 mL
1 tsp	cinnamon	5 mL

Preheat the oven to 325°F.

1. In a large bowl, use a fork to cream together the butter and brown sugar. Whip in the eggs and lemon zest and set aside.

2. In a medium-sized bowl, combine the flour with the baking powder.

3. In a small bowl, combine the streusel ingredients well with a fork or pastry cutter. Set aside.

4. Gradually add the flour and baking powder mixture in to the wet mixture and combine well with a wooden spoon. Spread this thick batter into a lightly buttered 9x13-inch baking dish. It will spread very thinly. Arrange the pear halves on top and press into the batter open-side down. Sprinkle the streusel evenly over the top and bake for approximately 1 hour or until a toothpick comes out of the center clean. Allow the cake to cool for 10 minutes before slicing.

— *Chloe Gregg*

" Sitting down at the table with old friends and new, nourishing them and being nouished by the deep intimacy that the Hollyhock atmosphere cultivates, adds another dimension to eating. Lingering over the gourmet food is one of Hollyhock's great pleasures."
— *Joan Borysenko*

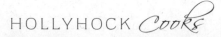

Pissaladière

This is pizza's elegant French cousin — a thin, crunchy crust is topped with sweet, caramelized onions, thyme and salty Romano cheese. For a delicious taste, add anchovies with the olives. These individual round "pizzas" can be a snack or a complete lunch.

1. In a large bowl, dissolve the honey in warm water, sprinkle in the yeast and allow it to stand until foamy, approximately 10 minutes.

2. Add the olive oil, salt, cornmeal and whole wheat flour to this sponge and stir well with a wooden spoon. Add the white flour until the dough is firm enough to handle and transfer it to a dry surface and knead in the remaining flour. Knead for approximately 10 minutes. Form the dough into a ball and set it in a lightly oiled bowl, cover with a damp towel and allow to rise in warm spot until doubled in size, about 1 hour.

3. In a large skillet, caramelize the onions in the olive oil until very soft and brown. Add the thyme and pepper and remove from the heat.

4. Preheat the oven to 400°F. Divide the dough into 8 small balls and use a rolling pin to roll each one out on a lightly floured surface until each one is quite thin and about 8 inches in diameter. Place each round on a lightly oiled baking sheet or parchment paper, with 4 rounds on each sheet. Sprinkle the cheese over each one and top with the onions and then the olive pieces. Bake for approximately 20 minutes or until the edges turn brown. Cool slightly on a cooling rack before serving.

— *Moreka Jolar*

Makes 8 pieces

DOUGH

1 cup	warm water	240 mL
1 tbsp	honey	15 mL
1 tbsp	active dry yeast	15 mL
3 tbsp	olive oil	45 mL
1 tsp	salt	5 mL
¼ cup	cornmeal	60 mL
1 cup	whole wheat flour	240 mL
1 cup	unbleached white flour	240 mL

TOPPING

3 tbsp	olive oil	45 mL
5 cups	thinly sliced yellow onions	1.2 L
2 tsp	chopped fresh thyme or 1 tsp dried	10 mL
1 tsp	black pepper	5 mL
2 cups	fresh grated Romano or mozzarella	480 mL
1 cup	coarsely chopped green or Kalamata olives	240 mL

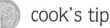 cook's tip

Using a very sharp knife when you are cutting onions is the best way to prevent burning "onion" eyes.

Pita Bread with Sesame Seeds

Fresh pita? What a treat. Dry, stale, store-bought pitas are not even in the same league.
Serve pita bread with just about anything, including Hummus (page 110),
Tzatziki (page 95) or White Bean Spread (page 112). Cut them into pockets and stuff
them with Tabouleh (page 27) or your favorite sandwich fillings.

Makes 1 dozen

1½ cups	warm water	360 mL
2 tbsp	honey	30 mL
2 tsp	active dry yeast	10 mL
3 tbsp	olive oil	45 mL
2 tbsp	unhulled sesame seeds	30 mL
1 tsp	salt	5 mL
1 cup	whole wheat flour	240 mL
1½ cups	unbleached white flour	360 mL

REQUIRES 2 LARGE BAKING SHEETS

 cook's tip

If you want the pita to puff up so that they can be easily cut into pockets, place the formed dough on a preheated baking sheet and then transfer immediately to the oven.

1. In a large bowl, dissolve the honey in the warm water and sprinkle the yeast over it. Allow it to stand for 15 minutes, or until the mixture is foamy.

2. Add the olive oil, seeds, salt and whole wheat flour and stir well with a wooden spoon. Gradually add the white flour until the dough is stiff enough to be transferred to a countertop and the remaining flour can be kneaded in. Knead for 5 minutes. Form the dough into a ball, place it in a lightly oiled bowl, and allow the dough to rise in a warm spot covered with a damp cloth for 1 hour, or until the dough doubles in size.

3. Preheat the oven to 400°F and preheat the baking sheets. Each baking sheet should be able to accommodate 4 to 6 pitas, but if you do not have large enough baking sheets, you can bake the pitas in batches. Punch the dough down and knead it a few times before dividing it into 12 equal pieces. Using a rolling pin and plenty of flour, roll each piece of dough into a round approximately 5 inches in diameter and place it on the baking sheets. Immediately place the baking sheets in the oven and bake until each pita is puffed up and browned. This will take approximately 15-20 minutes.

— *Moreka Jolar*

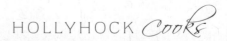

Roasted Garlic Focaccia with Dry Black Olives

You can't beat this classic Italian flatbread packed with rustic, dry black olives and bold, fresh rosemary. Topped with crisp roasted garlic, what more is left to desire? Perhaps a bowl of hot pasta on the side! You can also serve this focaccia fresh with small bowls of olive oil and balsamic vinegar, or slice it open and fill it with your favorite sandwich goodies.

1. In a large mixing bowl, dissolve the honey in the warm water and sprinkle in the yeast. Allow it to stand until the yeast is dissolved and foamy, approximately 15 minutes.

2. Add the chopped black olives, olive oil, chopped fresh rosemary, salt and whole wheat flour and mix well with a wooden spoon. Add the white flour until the dough is firm enough to handle with your hands and transfer it to a well-floured surface and knead in the remaining flour. Continue to knead for about 5 minutes. Transfer the dough to a large, lightly oiled bowl. Cover it tightly with plastic wrap or a damp cloth and put it in a warm spot until it doubles in size. This will take about 1½ hours.

3. Preheat the oven to 350°F. Punch the dough down and roll it out with a rolling pin to stretch out and evenly cover a lightly oiled baking sheet. Mix together the olive oil and the garlic for the topping and smear it evenly over the top of the dough. Sprinkle it with a small handful of rock salt and extra sprigs of rosemary if you like.

4. Bake for approximately 45 minutes, until bubbly and golden. Allow it to cool slightly on a cooling rack before cutting it into desired strips for serving.

VARIATION
As an alternative to olives, cut sundried tomatoes into strips and add them to dough.

* Dry-cured olives are available in most European delicatessens.

Moreka Jolar

Serves 10-15

DOUGH

2 cups	warm water	480 mL
¼ cup	honey	60 mL
2 tsp	active dry yeast	10 mL
1 cup	whole or chopped dry black olives *	240 mL
¼ cup	olive oil	60 mL
¼ cup	chopped fresh rosemary	60 mL
2 tsp	salt	10 mL
2 cups	whole wheat flour	480 mL
2½ cups	unbleached white flour	600 mL

TOPPING

10	cloves crushed garlic	10
¼ cup	olive oil	60 mL
	coarse rock salt	
	rosemary sprigs, if desired	

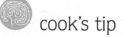 cook's tip

Leftover focaccia makes tasty croutons. Cut the bread into cubes, toss generously with olive oil and fresh oregano, lay on a baking sheet and bake at 250°F for as long as it takes to reach your desired level of crunchiness.

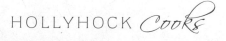

Roulade with Green Olive Tapenade

This is a bit like a savory cinnamon bun — a spiral of whole wheat dough layered with a spicy, green olive spread. It can be a decadent side dish to a pasta course or it can be a meal on its own. The tapenade is easy to prepare while the dough is rising.

Serves 6-8

1 batch	Green Olive Tapenade (page 109)	1 batch
1 cup	warm water	240 mL
1 tbsp	honey	15 mL
2 tsp	yeast	10 mL
2 tsp	salt	10 mL
1 cup	cold water	240 mL
2 cups	whole wheat flour	480 mL
5½ cups	unbleached white flour	1.3 L

1. In a large bowl, dissolve the honey in the warm water. Add the yeast and let stand for 10 minutes.

2. In a small cup, dissolve the salt in the cold water and add to the yeast mixture.

3. Use a wooden spoon to stir in the whole wheat flour. Begin to add the white flour, stirring well after each cup. When the dough is stiff enough to handle, transfer it to a dry surface and knead in the remaining flour. Knead for 15 minutes. When the dough is ready, you should be able to punch your fist in and bring it out clean. Shape the dough into a ball and let it rise in a lightly oiled bowl covered with plastic wrap or a damp cloth in a warm spot for approximately 1 hour or until it has doubled in size.

4. Use a rolling pin to roll out the dough into a rectangle that is about ¼-inch thick. Spread the Green Olive Tapenade evenly over the surface of the dough. Roll the length of the dough up as if you are rolling up cinnamon buns and pinch the seam where the dough meets. Use a sharp knife to cut 1-inch-thick rounds off this roll and lay these onto a lightly oiled baking sheet. Cover the rolls with a damp towel and let them rise for another hour.

5. Preheat the oven to 350°F. Bake the roulades for 30-45 minutes, until they are golden and firm through. Serve warm.

— *Moreka Jolar*

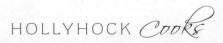

Savory Nut Tart Shell

This is a super-easy alternative to traditional pastry. It needs no rolling with a rolling pin, but is simply pressed into the bottom of the pan. The nuts give a crunchy texture and the paprika gives it a pleasing pink blush. Use it with Salmon Mousse Quiche (page 66) or Shrimp and Braised Leek Tart (page 68) or your favorite savory filling.

1. Process all the ingredients in a food processor until finely ground. Reserve 1 cup for your tart topping and gently press the remaining pastry into the bottom and sides of the tart or quiche pan. There is no need to pre-bake this pastry.

VARIATION
For a less rich pastry, substitute half of the ground nuts with ¼ cup of sunflower or pumpkin seeds.

— *Debra Fontaine*

Fills a 9-inch tart shell

1½ cups	flour	360 mL
½ cup	finely ground walnuts and/or almonds	120 mL
½ cup	soft butter	120 mL
½ tsp	paprika	2.5 mL
1½ tsp	salt	7.5 mL

"I enjoy the food at Hollyhock because it is beautiful and delicious, prepared with love, and served in a spectacular natural setting. I have very fond memories of meals on the deck at Hollyhock and look forward to more".
— Dr. Andrew Weil

Savory Zucchini Muffins

Anyone who grows zucchini is always looking for a way to creatively use up the bounty at harvest time. These muffins are moist, savory snacks that are packed with green zucchini goodness and topped with crisps of shredded Parmesan. These versatile muffins complement almost any soup or main dish.

Makes 1 dozen

2	eggs	2
¾ cup	milk	180 mL
⅔ cup	sunflower or safflower oil	160 mL
1½ cups	unbleached white flour	360 mL
1 cup	whole wheat flour	240 mL
¼ cup	brown sugar	60 mL
1 tbsp	baking powder	15 mL
1 tsp	salt	5 mL
2 cups	grated zucchini	480 mL
3 tbsp	chopped fresh basil	45 mL
½ cup	shredded Parmesan for topping	120 mL

Preheat the oven to 375°F.

1. In a large bowl, whisk together the eggs, milk and oil and set aside.

2. In a separate bowl, combine the flour with the brown sugar, baking powder and salt.

3. Add the grated zucchini and basil to the wet mixture. Use a wooden spoon to slowly mix the wet mixture into the dry mixture. Be careful not to over-mix; there should still be some lumps of flour remaining in the batter. Spoon the batter into lightly oiled muffin tins or muffin papers, and then top with the Parmesan and bake until brown, puffed, and firm to the touch, about 30-40 minutes.

VARIATION
Substitute a dairy alternative for the milk and omit the cheese to make non-dairy muffins.

— Moreka Jolar

" Here is the blessing I offer:
Earth, water, fire, air and
space combine to make
this food.
Numberless beings gave
their lives and labor
that we may eat.
May we be nourished
that we may nourish life. "
— Joan Halifax

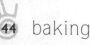

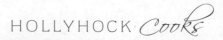

Spiced Carrot Muffins

For breakfast or a snack, these moist and low-fat muffins are filled with the sweet and irresistible spices of cinnamon, ginger, nutmeg and allspice. Slather these warm carrot muffins with one of Hollyhock's specialty butters (page 118).

Preheat the oven to 400°F.

1. In a small bowl, beat the eggs with a whisk and add the remaining wet ingredients including the grated carrot. Set aside.

2. In a large bowl, mix all the dry ingredients together well. Blend the wet mixture gently into the dry ingredients. Be careful not to over-mix; there should remain some lumps of flour in the batter. Divide the batter into the lightly oiled muffin tins or muffin papers. Bake for 18-25 minutes or until firm to the touch. Allow them to cool for 10 minutes before removing from them from the tins.

— Linda Gardner

Makes 1 dozen

4	eggs	4
½ cup	buttermilk	120 mL
1½ cups	grated carrot	360 mL
⅓ cup	oil	80 mL
1 tsp	vanilla extract	5 mL
1 cup	unbleached white flour	240 mL
½ cup	whole wheat flour	120 mL
½ cup	brown sugar	120 mL
2 tsp	baking powder	10 mL
1 tsp	baking soda	5 mL
1 tsp	cinnamon	5 mL
1 tsp	ginger	5 mL
½ tsp	salt	2.5 mL
½ tsp	nutmeg	2.5 mL
½ tsp	allspice	2.5 mL
½ cup	raisins or dried cranberries, if desired	120 mL

" The food at Hollyhock is an expression of the Beauty Path Way. It is always deliciously displayed and oh, so nurturing."
— Ann Mortifee

Spicy Cornmeal Muffins

Serve these excellent and easy cornmeal muffins with Black Bean Soup with Chipotle and Orange (page 34) or Fresh Green Soup (page 39). For a lighter muffin, substitute yogurt for the buttermilk and sour cream.

Makes 1 dozen

1 cup	buttermilk	240 mL
¼ cup	brown sugar	60 mL
¼ cup	sunflower or safflower oil	60 mL
¼ cup	sour cream	60 mL
1	egg	1
1¼ cups	whole wheat flour	300 mL
¾ cup	yellow cornmeal	180 mL
2 tsp	baking powder	30 mL
½ tsp	baking soda	2.5 mL
1 tbsp	diced fresh red or green chilis or half tbsp chili powder	15 mL
¼ cup	finely grated onions	60 mL
½ cup	finely chopped scallions	120 mL
½ cup	chopped fresh cilantro	120 mL
¾ cup	grated Monterey Jack cheese	180 mL

Preheat the oven to 400°F.

1. In a small bowl, whisk together the buttermilk with the brown sugar, oil, sour cream and egg. Set aside.

2. In a large bowl, combine the flour with cornmeal, baking powder and baking soda. Add the chopped fresh ingredients and the cheese to the dry mixture. Add all the wet ingredients to the dry and gradually mix. Be careful not to over-mix. Spoon the batter into lightly oiled muffin tins or muffin papers. Bake for 18-20 minutes until brown and firm to the touch. Allow them to cool for 5 minutes before lifting them out of the muffin tins.

— *Debra Fontaine*

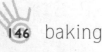
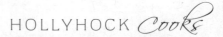
HOLLYHOCK *Cooks*

Spinach Feta Rolls

Rolled up like a savory cinnamon bun, this crunchy yeasted dough wraps around generous mounds of spinach and feta. Spinach feta rolls are like a meal on their own, with a distinctly Greek twist.

DOUGH

1. In a large bowl, dissolve the honey in the warm water and sprinkle in the yeast. Let it sit for 10 minutes, until foamy. Add the salt, semolina and whole wheat flour and stir well with a wooden spoon. Gradually add the white flour until the dough is stiff enough to handle. Transfer to a dry surface and knead in the remaining flour until you can punch your fist into the dough and bring it out clean. Shape the dough into a ball and place it in a lightly floured or oiled bowl, cover with a damp towel and allow it to rise in a warm spot for 1 hour, or until it has doubled in size.

FILLING

2. In a large skillet, sauté the onions, oregano and pepper until the onions are tender. Squeeze the excess water out of the spinach, add it to skillet and remove it from the heat.

3. Punch the dough down and use a rolling pin to roll it out on a lightly floured surface into a rectangle that is approximately ½-inch thick. Spread the spinach filling evenly over the surface of the dough, leaving half an inch of space around all the edges. Sprinkle the crumbled feta on top of the filling. Roll the length of the dough up as if you are making cinnamon buns and pinch the dough at the seam where it joins. Cut each spiral 1½-inches in width and place them on a lightly oiled baking sheet or parchment paper. Cover with a damp towel and let them rise for another 45 minutes.

4. Preheat the oven to 350°F. Bake for 1 hour, until golden and bubbly. Serve immediately or allow them to cool.

* Wheat semolina is the stuff with which one makes breakfast cream of wheat. It is available in the cereal sections of most stores.

— *Moreka Jolar*

Makes about 8 rolls

DOUGH

1 cup	warm water	240 mL
1 tbsp	honey	15 mL
1 tsp	yeast	5 mL
1 tsp	salt	5 mL
¼ cup	wheat semolina *	60 mL
1 cup	whole wheat flour	240 mL
2 cups	white flour	480 mL

FILLING

3 cups	diced onion	720 mL
2 tsp	chopped fresh oregano	10 mL
2 tsp	black pepper	10 mL
2 cups	steamed and chopped spinach	480 mL
1 cup	crumbled feta	240 mL

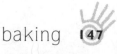

Zucchini Bread

Zucchinis the size of baseball bats come out of the earth on Cortes Island every summer, and once they start they just don't stop. If you ever wonder what to do with all that zucchini, here's a most delicious answer. This sweet, moist bread is ideal for breakfast, afternoon tea, or a light dessert.

Makes 1 loaf that serves 10-12

1½ cups	brown sugar	360 mL
¾ cup	sunflower or safflower oil	180 mL
3	eggs beaten	3
1½ tbsp	melted butter	23 mL
1 tsp	vanilla	5 mL
2 cups	grated zucchini	480 mL
1½ cups	unbleached white flour	360 mL
1 cup	whole wheat flour	240 mL
2 tsp	baking soda	10 mL
1 tsp	baking powder	5 mL
1 tsp	salt	5 mL
1 tsp	cinnamon	5 mL
1 tsp	ground cloves	5 mL
1 cup	roasted and chopped walnuts	240 mL

Preheat the oven to 350°F.

1. In a large bowl, combine the sugar, oil, eggs, butter and vanilla and beat well with a whisk. Mix in the grated zucchini.

2. In a separate bowl, combine all the remaining dry ingredients and mix well. Gently stir the dry mixture into the wet. Pour the batter into a well-oiled loaf pan and bake for approximately 1 hour, until firm and a toothpick comes out of the center clean. Cool for 15 minutes before removing from the pan.

— Linda Gardner

 cook's tip

If you are a sesame fan, try this: When baking loaves of sweet bread, line the oiled loaf pan with a thin layer of sesame seeds to help the loaf slip out after baking. This will also give the bread a crunchy sesame shell.

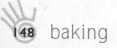

SEVEN

Desserts

WHEN HOLLYHOCK FIRST BEGAN, desserts weren't served at meals. But late at night, some of the founders were embarrassed to find that they were stealthily entering the kitchen and searching through the cabinets for something sweet. Self-denial, it was discovered, didn't work here. Thus sweet dishes found their rightful place on the Hollyhock table. All dinners now end in just the right place, with dessert. Once desserts were added to the dinner menu, sweet stuff started showing up other places too. Fresh baked cookies began to appear in a jar at the reception desk to greet weary travellers. And the skills of the cooks in the wonderful realm of the honeyed and sugary began to flow with fantastic results.

Desserts offer a beautiful canvas on which any cook can express his or her creativity. Desserts are a wonderful way to offer those you care about pure pleasure. For some people, dessert is the reason for eating in the first place. For others, dessert is a sweet indulgence, occasionally taken and greatly appreciated. For a few, they're a stolen pleasure. Our dessert selection includes something for the calorie conscious, much for the careful connoisseur, and a great deal for unabashedly enthusiastic.

A chocolate dessert provides a delicious end to a Mexican meal. Lemon squares offer a graceful denouement to a seafood feast. With a heavy, cheesy entrée, a fruity dessert like a pie or a crisp lifts the meal to higher heights. Sometimes simply fresh fruit will suffice. Many will agree: it is an act of great loving kindness to serve homemade dessert at the end of a meal.

Almond Biscotti with Fennel and Black Pepper

Here is a new spin on a classic Italian cookie. There is just enough black pepper in this recipe to give these sweet biscuits a provocative spice. Drizzle these delicious cookies with melted white chocolate for a decadent treat. Dunk them in Chai (page 192) or Mexican Hot Chocolate (page 195) on another occasion.

Makes 1 dozen

2¾ cups	unbleached white flour	660 mL
1 cup	sugar	240 mL
1 cup	slivered almonds	240 mL
1 tbsp	whole fennel seeds	15 mL
2 tsp	baking powder	10 mL
1 tsp	black pepper	5 mL
	pinch of salt	
4	eggs	4
¼ cup	sunflower or safflower oil	60 mL
1 tsp	almond extract	5 mL

Preheat the oven to 350°F.

1. In a large bowl, combine all the dry ingredients together except for ½ cup of the slivered almonds, which should be reserved for the topping.

2. In a separate small bowl, combine the eggs, oil and almond extract with a whisk.

3. Add the wet ingredients to the dry. Mix and knead with your hands until the dough comes together well. Turn the dough onto a lightly oiled baking sheet and use your hands to form it into a log, approximately 4x13 inches. Wet your hands slightly to avoid stickiness while you are shaping the dough.

4. Cover the log with the remaining half a cup of slivered almonds and gently press them into the top and sides of the dough. Bake for 30-40 minutes. Remove from the oven and then use 2 spatulas to gently lift the log onto a cooling rack. Allow it to cool for 20 minutes. Slice the log into diagonal cookies, approximately 1 inch in width. Lay each one down on the baking sheet and re-bake for another 20 minutes. Turn the oven off, open the oven door a crack and allow the biscotti to cool in the oven. This will help them to crisp up a little more. They will keep in a sealed container for up to 2 weeks or frozen for up to 2 months.

— *Moreka Jolar*

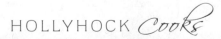

Apple Berry Pie

This pie's pastry is fluffy and light with a melt-in-your-mouth texture. The apple and berry filling will bring the sweet taste of summer to your plate, no matter what the season. Serve topped with vanilla ice cream or whipped cream.

Preheat the oven to 350°F.

1. In a large bowl, combine the apples with the lemon juice. Add the berries to the apple and sprinkle with flour, sweetener and cinnamon and combine well.

2. Divide the prepared and chilled pastry into 2 portions. Use a rolling pin to roll out 1 portion of the pastry on a lightly floured surface until it is big enough that it will fit the bottom and sides of the pie dish. It will be about a ¼-inch thick. Wrap the prepared pastry around the rolling pin and lift and lay into the pie dish. Trim the edges to fit the pie dish. Fill the pie dish with the prepared filling.

3. Roll out the second portion of pastry and lay it out on top of the filling. Trim to fit and pinch the edges together where the pastry meets. Score the top a few times with a fork. Bake for 45 minutes, until the top pastry is golden. Allow the pie to cool for 20 minutes before serving, or serve later at room temperature.

* See page 123 for instructions.

— *Moreka Jolar*

Serves 8-10

1 batch	Double Crust Basic Whole Wheat Pastry *	1 batch
2	large thinly sliced crisp apples	2
	juice of 1 lemon	
2 cups	fresh or partially thawed berries such as blueberries, raspberries, loganberries, huckleberries or blackberries	480 mL
¼ cup	white or whole wheat flour	60 mL
¼ cup	sugar or honey	60 mL
2 tsp	cinnamon	10 mL

Requires a deep 9-inch pie dish

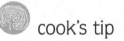 cook's tip

Be careful to handle pastry as little as possible while preparing it. Pastry does not like to be kneaded. The less you handle the pastry, the lighter and flakier the end result will be. It takes some practice — be patient with yourself.

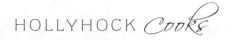 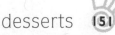

Blackberries
with Honey-Lavender Custard

Blackberries and lavender meet in this silky, fragrant and rich dessert. It can be served warm or cold. Garnish this refined dessert with sprigs of fresh lavender.

Serves 8-10

4 cups	heavy cream	960 mL
2 tbsp	fresh lavender flowers	30 mL
8	egg yolks	8
½ cup	liquid honey	120 mL
8-10 cups	blackberries or raspberries	2-2.5 L

REQUIRES 8-10 OVENPROOF DISHES OR RAMEKINS

 cook's tip

There's nothing worse than curdled custard. To avoid curdling, have a small bowl of ice cubes standing by while you prepare any custard. As soon as you see the signs of curdling, remove from the heat immediately and whisk in 1 ice cube. This will usually remedy the situation.

1. In a small saucepan, combine the heavy cream and lavender and simmer for 10-20 minutes, until the lavender flavor infuses the cream. Be careful not to boil it.

2. In a large bowl, whisk the egg yolks with the honey until well combined. Add a small amount of the warm cream to the egg yolks, whisking constantly. Do not add all the cream at once or you could curdle the eggs. Whisk in the rest of the cream to this mixture.

3. Return the mixture to the saucepan. Cook over low heat, stirring constantly, until the mixture thickens enough to coat the back of a wooden spoon. Continue to be careful not to let this custard boil or it will curdle.

4. Remove the custard from the heat and pour it through a fine strainer and into a small stainless steel bowl to remove the lavender flowers. Set this bowl into a larger bowl of ice and chill for 30 minutes.

5. Preheat the broiler. Divide the berries between 8 to 10 lightly oiled ramekins or small ovenproof dishes. Top with the custard. Broil for 2-3 minutes, until the top of the custard bubbles and browns slightly. Serve warm or chilled.

— Carmen Rosse

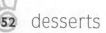

Brownie Pudding Cake

Little is required to concoct this simple and gooey chocolate treat. A spoon, a whisk and a little time is all you need for this brownie gone wild.

Preheat the oven to 350°F.

STEP ONE

1. Lightly oil a 9x9-inch baking pan. In a small bowl, combine the brown sugar and cocoa and sprinkle the mixture into the bottom of the baking pan. Pour the hot water over this and mix gently with a wooden spoon. The consistency will be lumpy.

STEP TWO

2. In a medium-sized mixing bowl, combine the flour, cocoa powder, baking powder and salt.

3. In a separate small bowl, beat the egg. Mix in the brown sugar, melted butter and vanilla. Add the dry ingredients to the wet and mix well with a wooden spoon or whisk, until there are no lumps in the batter. Add the nuts now, if desired.

4. Drop spoonfuls of the batter evenly into the mixture of cocoa powder and brown sugar, which is already covering the bottom of the pan. Bake for 35 minutes. Let the cake sit for 20 minutes to allow the pudding to set before serving. It can be served warm, or refrigerated and served chilled.

— *Dianne West*

Serves 10-12

STEP ONE

⅔ cups	brown sugar	160 mL
3 tbsp	cocoa powder, if possible Dutch	45 mL
1½ cups	hot water	360 mL

STEP TWO

⅓ cup	unbleached white flour	80 mL
2 tbsp	cocoa powder	30 mL
¼ tsp	baking powder	1.2 mL
⅛ tsp	salt	0.5 mL
1	egg	1
½ cup	brown sugar	120 mL
2 tbsp	melted butter	30 mL
1 tsp	vanilla	5 mL
¼ cup	diced walnuts, if desired	60 mL

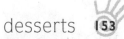

Banana-Berry Ice

This is a quick, simple way to make an ice-cream-like dessert that is all fruit and has few calories. The bananas give it a rich creamy texture. Serve it in cups, glasses or bowls.

Serves 8-10

4	frozen bananas	4
	zest and juice of 1 lime	
2 cups	frozen raspberries or strawberries	480 mL

cook's tip

Freeze bananas in their skins. This minimizes the natural browning that occurs with peeled bananas. Before use, simply run the banana under hot water for a minute or so until it easily slips out of the skin.

1. Place the frozen bananas, lime zest and juice in a food processor and process until soft and creamy, about 2 minutes. You may need to allow them to thaw slightly before processing.

2. Add the frozen berries and process for another minute or so until the mixture turns bright pink. Serve immediately or re-freeze for up to 1 month. Garnish with fresh berries, toasted coconut or dark chocolate sauce.

VARIATIONS
Try adding 1 cup of coconut cream or heavy cream to the bananas while processing for a richer and more decadent dessert.

— *Moreka Jolar*

Cheesecake Sauce for Fresh Fruit

Inspired by a cheesecake craving, this sauce was invented one hot summer day when berries were in season. Here is instant cheesecake flavor without turning on your oven. This sauce keeps well in the refrigerator for at least a week. It's particularly good on berries, so make a double batch to have on hand for instant gratification. Warning — highly addictive!

Makes 2 cups

9 oz.	Philadelphia-style cream cheese at room temperature	260 g
9 oz.	sour cream	260 g
2 tbsp	fresh lemon juice	30 mL
4 tbsp	white sugar	60 mL
½ tsp	vanilla	2.5 mL

1. In a food processor or mixing bowl, blend the cream cheese until soft. Add the sour cream and continue to blend until the 2 are well mixed. Add the lemon juice, sugar and vanilla and blend. Refrigerate. Serve chilled over fresh berries or tropical fruits.

— *Hanyu Wasyliw*

Chocolate Bottom Banana Cream Pie

The bottom pastry of this pie is covered with a perfect, thin layer of chocolate, which is then topped off with bananas and smooth, creamy custard. A mountain of whipped cream finishes off the whole affair. Food fit for angels.

1. Cook the single pie crust according to the instructions on page 123.

2. In a heavy saucepan, whisk together the sugar and cornstarch. Add just enough milk to whisk this into a smooth paste in order to dissolve the cornstarch. Continue to add the remaining milk.

3. In a small bowl, beat the egg yolks and then whisk them into the milk mixture. Gently heat on medium, stirring with the whisk, until the custard begins to thicken and then lower the heat. Continue to cook for about 10-15 minutes on low heat stirring constantly until the custard is thick like a pudding. Remove from heat. Whisk in the vanilla and set aside.

4. Use a double boiler to gently heat ¼ cup of milk with the chocolate until it is completely melted. Spread this evenly into the pre-baked and cooled pie shell.

5. Arrange the sliced bananas over the chocolate and top with the custard. Chill for at least 4 hours. Before serving, whip the cream with some sweetener if you like. Spread the whipped cream over the custard.

* You can use the remaining 6 egg whites to make two batches of pavlovas (page 170).

— Moreka Jolar

Serves 8-10

1	Single Crust Basic Whole Wheat Pastry	1
½ cup	sugar	120 mL
3 tbsp	cornstarch	45 mL
2¾ cups	milk or soy milk	660 mL
6	egg yolks *	6
1 tsp	vanilla extract	5 mL
4 oz.	dark chocolate or ¾ cup chocolate chips	115 g
3	bananas sliced in rounds	3
2 cups	heavy cream	480 mL

REQUIRES A DEEP 9-INCH PIE PAN

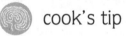 cook's tip

If you don't have a double boiler, you can make one by simply resting a small stainless steel bowl into the top of a saucepan.

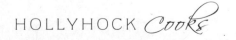 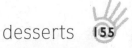

Chocolate Oatmeal Cookies with Orange

These hearty, whole wheat cookies are moist and infused with the vibrant tang of fresh orange zest. This batter will keep refrigerated for up to one month or for three months frozen.

Makes 2 dozen

I cup	soft butter	240 mL
½ cup	brown sugar	120 mL
2	eggs	2
2 tbsp	orange zest	30 mL
I tsp	vanilla	5 mL
1½ cups	chopped nuts such as almonds, walnuts or hazelnuts	360 mL
1½ cups	chocolate chips	360 mL
I cup	oats	240 mL
I cup	shredded coconut	240 mL
1½ cups	whole wheat or spelt flour	360 mL
I tbsp	cinnamon	15 mL
I tsp	baking soda	5 mL

Preheat the oven to 300 °F.

1. In a large bowl, use a fork to cream together the butter and sugar. Add the eggs, orange zest and vanilla and continue to mix. Mix in the nuts, chocolate chips, oats and coconut.

2. In a separate bowl, combine together the flour, cinnamon, and baking soda. Gradually add the flour mixture to the wet mixture and stir well with your hands or with a wooden spoon.

3. Shape the dough into balls and place them on a lightly oiled cookie sheet or parchment paper and press down with a fork. Bake for 15 minutes, just until golden for a soft and chewy cookie or longer for a crisper cookie.

— *Linda Gardner*

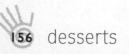 cook's tip

Always use organic fruit when using the zest of citrus. If this is not available, be sure to wash the fruit well with hot soapy water before using.

 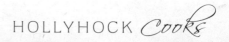

Chocolate Tofu Cheesecake

This dense and silky cake needs a minimum of two hours refrigeration time before serving, but it is most delectable when refrigerated overnight. With two hours of refrigeration, the cake has a slightly crumbly texture that is mitigated by its lush, rich chocolate presentation. Dress the cake up with a coating of toasted slivered almonds covering the top, or with thinly sliced apricots, peaches, strawberries, blueberries or edible flowers.

Preheat the oven to 350°F.

1. In a small bowl, combine the graham cracker crumbs and melted butter or oil and press evenly into the greased bottom of a 10-inch springform pan. Bake the graham cracker crust at 350°F for 15 minutes, or until it begins to turn golden. Remove from the oven and set aside.

2. Put the tofu into a food processor with the vanilla extract. Blend for about 2 minutes or until no more chunks are left in the tofu and the texture becomes totally smooth. Leave in the food processor.

3. Divide the chocolate into 5 to 10 chunks and place them in a double boiler. Heat the chocolate at a low temperature until it is fully melted. Add it to the tofu in the food processor and mix them together until they are completely smooth. This should take about 4 minutes of mixing.

4. Using a rubber spatula, pour the tofu-chocolate mixture over the crust. Bake the cheesecake for 40 minutes or until a knife comes out of the center of the cake clean. Refrigerate for a minimum of 2 hours before serving.

— *Moreka Jolar*

Serves 12-16

2 cups	crushed graham crackers	480 mL
¾ cup	melted butter, or sunflower or safflower oil	180 mL
25 oz.	extra-firm silken-style tofu	715 g
15 oz.	semi-sweet dark chocolate	430 g
2 tsp	vanilla extract	10 mL
1 tsp	almond extract or 1 tbsp (15 mL) orange zest, if desired	5 mL

REQUIRES A 10-INCH SPRINGFORM PAN

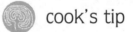 cook's tip

Use "real" vanilla extract. Artificial vanilla extract may pose as a worthy substitute, but don't be fooled. The dish is as good as the ingredients you put into it.

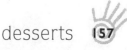

Chocolate Tofu Pudding

This non-dairy pudding is low in fat but rich in flavor.
It is simple to make and has a silky smooth texture.

Serves 2

12 oz.	firm silken-style tofu	340 g
1 tsp	vanilla extract	5 mL
4 oz.	semi-sweet dark chocolate or ¾ cup chocolate chips	115 g

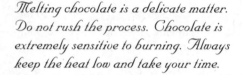 **cook's tip**

Melting chocolate is a delicate matter. Do not rush the process. Chocolate is extremely sensitive to burning. Always keep the heat low and take your time.

1. Process the tofu and vanilla in a food processor for about 2 minutes, until smooth.

2. Use a double boiler to gently melt the chocolate. Keep it on medium heat and stir often with a wooden spoon.

3. Add the warm, melted chocolate to the tofu in the food processor and continue to process for another 2 minutes, until the pudding is completely silky and smooth. Serve immediately or, for a more firm dessert, chill the pudding for 1 hour.

VARIATIONS

For a richer and thicker pudding, melt another 2 ounces of chocolate. For other variations, try adding ½ tsp almond extract, 2 tsp orange zest or 1 tsp ground cardamom as you process the pudding. For other options, fold in a handful of sliced candied ginger, banana, berries or toasted coconut.

— *Moreka Jolar*

HOLLYHOCK *Cooks*

Cocoa Banana Cake

This moist, dense cake uses bananas as a sweetener, keeping it rich but
low in fat. Purée the bananas in a food processor or with a potato masher and
delight in the marriage of banana and chocolate. Topped with the cocoa
banana frosting, it's an outstanding treat. If you love nuts, fold half a cup of
chopped walnuts into the batter.

Preheat the oven to 350°F.

1. In a measuring cup, combine the milk with the vinegar and set aside.

2. In a large bowl, cream together the butter and brown sugar. Add the
   eggs, banana purée and vanilla and mix well.

3. In a separate bowl, combine all the remaining dry ingredients. Use a
   wooden spoon to stir the dry ingredients slowly into the wet mixture.
   Be careful not to over-mix the batter or the cake will turn doughy.
   The batter can remain a bit lumpy.

4. Spoon the batter into a well-oiled Bundt pan. Bake for 40-45 minutes,
   until a wooden skewer comes out of the center clean. Allow it to cool for
   10 minutes before running a knife along all the edges and inverting the
   cake onto a cooling rack. When the cake is completely cool, ice it with
   Cocoa Banana Frosting (below) or Chocolate Tofu Pudding (page 158).

— *Anne Pitman*

Serves 12-16

⅔ cup	milk	160 mL
1 tbsp	vinegar	15 mL
1 cup	soft butter	240 mL
1⅓ cups	brown sugar	320 mL
2	eggs beaten	2
1½ cups	puréed banana	360 mL
2 tsp	vanilla extract	10 mL
2 cups	unbleached white flour	480 mL
1 cup	cocoa powder	240 mL
1½ tsp	baking powder	7.5 mL
1 tsp	baking soda	5 mL
½ tsp	salt	2.5 mL

REQUIRES 1 BUNDT PAN

Cocoa Banana Frosting

The banana keeps this icing silky and moist. If you have a food processor,
start by pureeing the banana and then add the remaining ingredients.
A potato masher and a strong arm will do the trick too.

1. In a medium-sized bowl or food processor, mix together the cocoa
   powder, butter, banana, milk and vanilla. While whisking or mixing, slowly
   add the icing sugar and continue to work with the whisk, electric mixer,
   or food processor until smooth.

— *Anne Pitman*

Makes about 3 cups

½ cup	sifted cocoa powder	120 mL
¼ cup	melted butter	60 mL
¼ cup	puréed banana	60 mL
2 tbsp	milk	30 mL
½ tsp	vanilla extract	2.5 mL
3 cups	sifted confectioners sugar	720 mL

Coconut Carrot Macaroons

Finally, vegans rejoice! This macaroon recipe ingeniously uses sticky honey instead of egg to hold it all together. Carrot keeps these macaroons healthful, moist and not too sweet. If you're looking for a sweet that isn't too sweet, here's your recipe.

Makes 1 dozen

1 cup	grated carrots	240 mL
1 cup	shredded coconut	240 mL
½ cup	honey	120 mL
⅓ cup	sunflower or safflower oil	80 mL
1 cup	unbleached white flour	240 mL
1 tsp	baking powder	5 mL
1 tsp	cinnamon	5 mL

Preheat the oven to 350°F.

1. In a large bowl, combine the carrots and coconut with the honey and oil.

2. In a separate bowl, mix the flour with the baking powder and cinnamon. Add the flour mixture to the wet mixture and combine completely with your hands or a wooden spoon.

3. Spoon the batter in 12 equal portions onto a lightly oiled baking sheet or parchment paper. Bake for 25 minutes, until firm to the touch. Allow them to cool on a cooling rack.

— *Annie Brae*

cook's tip

If you measure the oil first and then the honey, the honey will slip right out of the measuring cup.

Coconut Tapioca

Make this sweet, creamy pudding your own by altering its toppings or ingredients. Use less sweetener, if preferred, or sweeten it by adding two diced bananas to the tapioca while cooking. Use soy milk with half the coconut milk for a less rich dessert. Top with toasted coconut, fresh mango, pineapple or strawberries.

Serves 6-8

4 cups	coconut milk	960 mL
8 tbsp	non-instant tapioca pearls	120 mL
½ cup	sweetener such as honey or maple syrup	120 mL

1. In a small saucepan, mix the coconut milk with the tapioca pearls and let them stand for 20 minutes.

2. Stir in the sweetener and begin to heat very slowly. Use a heat diffuser if you have one.

3. Continue to heat on low for 1 hour, stirring often, until the pearls are transparent. Be careful not to allow this to boil. Remove from heat. Serve immediately or at room temperature.

— *Moreka Jolar*

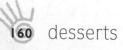

Cream Puffs

Do not be intimidated by how gorgeous and impressive these cream puffs look when served. A beginner cook can easily make them. This recipe will yield a light, flaky pastry every time. Speed is the key. Have the baking sheets ready and the oven hot as soon as this batter is done. When the puffs are cool and ready for filling, we've given you a few ideas for fillings.

Preheat the oven to 400°F.

1. Before you get started, it is important to note that this batter shouldn't sit at all. It must go immediately from the saucepan, to the baking sheet, to the hot oven. In a medium-sized saucepan, heat the water and butter until it comes to a rolling boil and the butter is melted.

2. Remove from the heat and vigorously whisk in the flour. When the flour is entirely mixed in, add the eggs, 1 at a time, whisking well between each one. Beat well until you have a gluey batter. An electric mixer is ideal for this.

3. Immediately spoon the batter in ice-cream-scoop-sized balls onto parchment paper on baking sheets and bake until each puff is very golden and puffed, about 20-30 minutes. When the puffs are done baking, turn the oven off and leave the oven door slightly ajar but leave puffs in the oven until cool. This ensures they do not fall.

4. When completely cool, use a knife to cut a small slice in the side of each puff and fill with your choice of filling. If sweet, garnish with icing sugar or chocolate sauce, and serve immediately.

VARIATIONS

Here are some ideas for fillings

- 3 cups (720 mL) heavy cream whipped and folded with fresh berries
- Your favorite chilled custard
- 2 batches of Chocolate Tofu Pudding (page 158)
- Savory fillings such as crab salad are also great.

— *Debra Fontaine*

Makes about 10-12

1 cup	water	240 mL
½ cup	butter	120 mL
1 cup	unbleached white flour	240 mL
4	eggs	4

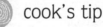 cook's tip

This recipe can be easily multiplied to feed a large crowd. Just be sure you have the oven space for the entire recipe to fit in all at once, as the puffs have to bake at the same time and be allowed to cool in the oven to ensure that they do not fall.

 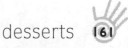

Dream Bars

Eat up and dream on. Dream bars are a snap to make and are favorite treats at Hollyhock.
The top layer of the bar is chock-full of healthy items such as nuts, raisins, and oats,
along with decadent chocolate chips. Sunflower or pumpkin seeds can be used as
an alternative to nuts if you like.

Serves 10-12

CRUST

1 cup	unbleached white flour	240 mL
½ cup	soft butter	120 mL
2 tbsp	brown sugar	30 mL

TOPPING

1 cup	brown sugar	240 mL
½ cup	whole rolled oats	120 mL
½ cup	shredded coconut	120 mL
½ cup	raisins	120 mL
½ cup	chopped mixed nuts such as almonds, hazelnut or walnuts	120 mL
½ cup	chocolate chips	120 mL
3	eggs beaten	3
1 tsp	vanilla extract	5 mL

Preheat the oven to 350°F.

1. In a small bowl, use a fork to combine the crust ingredients and press the mixture into the bottom of a lightly oiled, 8-inch square or round baking dish. Bake for 15 minutes.

2. Meanwhile, in a large bowl, combine all the topping ingredients and mix them well. Pour over the partially baked crust and bake for another 15-20 minutes. Allow it to cool completely before cutting into bars.

— *Linda Gardner*

"*The most important blessing I can think of before eating is the simple act of being present. It's so easy to rush to the table and devour your food while being everywhere but there. Who wants to eat your errands, your income taxes or your e-mails? By centering on the breath for even two or three cycles I come back home to myself, and can bring my attention more fully to the gift of taste, nourishment and abundance which is so easy to take for granted.*"
— *Joan Borysenko*

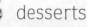

HOLLYHOCK *Cooks*

Fruit Turnovers with Ginger and Cardamom

These dainty turnovers are made of rich and flaky pastry wrapped around soft, baked fruit and ginger. They are a welcome addition to breakfast as well as afternoon tea.

Preheat the oven to 350°F.

1. Combine the fruit with the lemon juice, ginger, cinnamon, cardamom and nutmeg and set the mixture aside.

2. Pile the 4 sheets of filo on a dry surface. Use sharp scissors to cut down the center in each direction of the pile, making four squares out of each piece, giving 16 pieces in total. Each turnover uses 2 squares of filo.

3. Mix the vanilla into the melted butter and brush it lightly over one square. Place 1 cup of fruit filling at the bottom and, lifting up 2 layers of pastry, roll it up like you are wrapping a burrito, buttering each side as you roll. Tuck the ends under and place on a baking sheet. Continue this process until all 8 turnovers are done. Bake at 350°F for 1 hour, until turnovers are golden and crispy. Serve immediately.

VARIATIONS

Try using peaches, plums or mangoes in place of the banana. For extra sweetness, you can also sprinkle the turnovers with brown sugar before baking. To reheat any leftover pastries, simply place them back in the oven at 350°F for 10-20 minutes and they will become crispy again.

— *Annabel Davis*

Serves 8

4	sheets filo pastry	4
4 cups	thinly sliced apples	960 mL
4 cups	diced bananas	960 mL
	juice of 1 lemon	
1½ tbsp	freshly grated ginger	23 mL
1 tsp	cinnamon	5 mL
¾ tsp	ground cardamom	4 mL
¾ tsp	ground nutmeg	4 mL
½ cup	melted butter	120 mL
1 tsp	vanilla extract	5 mL

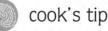 cook's tip

Keep the filo pastry moist. Use it immediately after unwrapping it or cover it with a slightly damp towel until you are ready to use it. Re-seal the remaining pastry with plastic wrap. It keeps well when frozen, too.

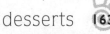

Gingerbread Cake

Imagine waking up to the smell of fresh gingerbread wafting out of the kitchen. This is a wonderful breakfast cake that can also be served for dessert. This dark, moist cake is packed with the taste of fresh ginger. Top it with some apple sauce for a breakfast treat, or with ice cream for dessert.

Serves 10-12

½ cup	soft butter	120 mL
½ cup	brown sugar	120 mL
I	egg	I
½ cup	unsulphured molasses	120 mL
½ cup	finely grated fresh ginger	120 mL
2 tsp	vanilla extract	10 mL
½ cup	milk	120 mL
I tbsp	vinegar	15 mL
I cup	whole wheat flour	240 mL
I cup	unbleached white flour	240 mL
I tsp	baking soda	5 mL
½ tsp	salt	2.5 mL

REQUIRES A 10-INCH SPRINGFORM PAN

 cook's tip

Always sift the baking soda and baking powder when baking. They are often full of little hard lumps and there's nothing worse then finding a bitter lump in your cake.

Preheat the oven to 350°F.

1. In a large bowl, use a fork to cream together the butter and sugar. Whisk in the egg, molasses, ginger and vanilla extract.

2. In a small bowl, combine the milk with the vinegar. Add this to the wet mixture.

3. In a third bowl, combine all the remaining dry ingredients. Slowly stir the dry mixture into the wet with a wooden spoon just until they are completely combined. Pour the batter into a lightly oiled 10-inch springform pan and bake for 30-35 minutes, or until a knife comes out of the center clean. Allow it to cool slightly before removing. Serve warm topped with whipped cream or apple sauce.

— *Moreka Jolar*

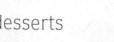
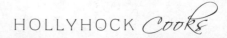

Killer Peanut Butter Fudge Cookies

Packed with peanut butter and dark fudge, these chewy cookies won't kill you,
but you might think you've gone to heaven for a while.

Preheat the oven to 350°F.

1. In a medium-sized bowl, use a fork to cream together the peanut butter, oil, sugars, eggs and vanilla.

2. In another bowl, mix together the remaining dry ingredients.

3. Add the dry ingredients one-half at a time to the creamed ingredients and mix well. The dough will be stiff, so this is easiest done with lightly oiled hands.

4. Roll heaping tablespoons of dough by hand into 1 to 1½-inch balls. Place them on lightly oiled baking sheets 3 inches apart. Flatten each ball with a fork. Bake for 8-10 minutes. Allow the cookies to cool slightly on the baking sheet before transferring to a cooling rack.

— *Carmen Rosse*

Makes 24 cookies

1 cup	peanut butter	240 mL
⅓ cup	vegetable oil	80 mL
1 cup	white sugar	240 mL
1 cup	packed brown sugar	240 mL
2	eggs beaten	2
1 tsp	vanilla extract	5 mL
⅔ cup	cocoa powder	160 mL
1 cup	unbleached white flour	240 mL
1 tsp	baking soda	5 mL
½ tsp	salt	2.5 mL

" Hollyhock food is the most exquisite, nourishing, fresh, eclectic food imaginable. When the bell rings to announce a meal, priorities are shuffled, and all bodies head for the lodge, to taste the latest magic betwixt cooks and gardens, land and sea. In a place this beautiful, with people and work and play this absorbing, only incredible food would pull us all together in solidarity for chowing down. "
— *Gregor Robertson*

Layered Nut Torte

This easy to prepare torte is bursting with rich nutty taste. The fun comes when you slice the cake into layers and fill and top this torte with whatever your creative heart desires. We've given you a few ideas and guidelines below. Keep it simple or cover it with whipped cream, rose petals and fresh fruit. This stunning celebratory cake is great for occasions ranging from weddings to births.

Serves 12-16

12	eggs	12
2 cups	white sugar	480 mL
2 tsp	vanilla extract	10 mL
3 cups	toasted and finely ground hazelnuts or almonds	720 mL
1 cup	unbleached white flour	240 mL
1 tsp	baking powder	5 mL
½ tsp	salt	2.5 mL

REQUIRES A 9-INCH SPRINGFORM PAN

cook's tip

Fishing line or any other firm nylon string is great for evenly slicing layers of a cake. Hold the piece of line tightly between your hands and run it through the cake.

Preheat the oven to 350°F.

1. Lightly oil a 9-inch springform pan and dust with a thin layer of flour.

2. Separate the eggs and reserve the egg whites in the fridge.

3. In a large bowl, beat the egg yolks and sugar with a whisk until thick and foamy. Whisk in the vanilla.

4. In a separate bowl, combine the ground nuts, flour, baking powder and salt.

5. In a large, dry bowl, beat the egg whites until they form stiff peaks.

6. Add the dry mixture to the mixture of egg yolks and sugar and combine well with a wooden spoon. Fold in the beaten egg whites until well combined. Immediately pour the batter into the springform pan. Bake for 40-50 minutes, until the torte is brown and beginning to puff up in the center. A toothpick should come out of the center clean. Allow it to cool completely on a cooling rack before removing from the pan.

7. Use a sharp bread knife to slice the torte into 2 layers. Fill and dress with your favorite combination and serve.

FILLING AND TOPPING IDEAS

• Spread a thin layer of fresh fruit or sauce between the tortes and cover the entire cake with 3 cups (720 mL) heavy cream, whipped.

• Two batches of Chocolate Tofu Pudding (page 158) combined with 3 tbsp (45 mL) of instant coffee granules.

• One batch Cocoa Banana Frosting (page 159).

• Fill with fresh berries and cover with Cheesecake Sauce (page 154).

— *Shivon Robinsong*

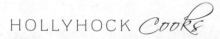

Lemon Squares

These lemon squares are a sinful pleasure. A rich and flaky shortbread crust is topped with silky, firm and tart lemon custard. If you are going to go decadent, go all the way.

Preheat the oven to 350°F

1. Over medium heat, toast the almonds in a heavy, ungreased skillet, stirring them often until they are golden brown. Grind them in a food processor. Process the ground almonds and the rest of the crust ingredients in a food processor by pulsing them until crumbly. Pat this into a greased 9x13-inch baking dish and bake for 18-20 min, until golden. Allow the crust to cool for 15-20 minutes.

2. In a medium-sized bowl, beat the eggs, egg yolks and sugar together with a whisk until smooth. Whisk in the lemon juice and then sprinkle the flour in using the whisk to prevent lumps of flour in the mixture. Pour this mixture over the baked crust and bake for 40 minutes. Cool on rack and then chill in the fridge for at least 2 hours before slicing.

— *Debra Fontaine*

 cook's tip

When slicing chilled custard bars such as these, run the knife under hot water first to achieve a nice clean cut.

Makes 16-20 squares

CRUST		
¾ cup	unbleached white flour	180 mL
¾ cup	toasted, ground almonds	180 mL
¾ tbsp	white sugar	90 mL
¾ cup	soft butter	180 mL

TOPPING		
5	large eggs	5
2	egg yolks	2
2¼ cups	white sugar	540 mL
1 cup	freshly squeezed lemon juice	240 mL
¼ cup	unbleached white flour	60 mL

Mango Fool

Raspberries or strawberries also make lovely "fools." Use about two cups of fruit purée to one cup of heavy cream. Layering golden mango fool with rosy raspberry or strawberry fool in a wine glass makes a simple, but spectacular summer dessert. You can also use this fool to fill cream puffs (page 161).

1. Peel the mangoes and cut the flesh off the pit. Purée the flesh in a food processor.

2. In a medium-sized bowl, whip the cream and sugar. Fold in the mango purée. Spoon the fool into parfait or wine glasses. Garnish with a sprig of mint or a few fresh berries. Chill for an hour before serving.

— *Hanyu Wasyliw*

Serves 4

2	ripe mangoes	2
1 cup	heavy cream	250 mL
1 tbsp	white sugar	15 mL

 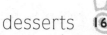

Mango Ginger Upside-Down Cake

The mango baked with sugar gives this cake a caramel-like top that turns it into a gooey extravaganza. Candied ginger bits throughout the cake spice up each sweet bite. This is a must for anyone who loves the idea of upside-down cake and who is wild about mangoes. Who isn't?

Serves 8-10

2	ripe mangoes	2
¾ cup	melted butter	180 mL
1 tbsp	freshly grated ginger	15 mL
1¼ cups	brown sugar	300 mL
¾ cup	soft butter	180 mL
2 tsp	vanilla extract	10 mL
3	eggs	3
½ cup	yogurt	120 mL
½ cup	wheat semolina	120 mL
⅓ cup	finely sliced candied ginger	80 mL
1 cup	unbleached white flour	240 mL
2 tsp	baking powder	10 mL
½ tsp	cinnamon	2.5 mL

REQUIRES 1 DEEP 9-INCH PIE PLATE

Preheat the oven to 350°F.

1. Peel the mangoes, cut away the pits, and slice the flesh into thin strips. Arrange the strips of fruit in the bottom of an ungreased, deep, 9-inch pie plate.

2. In a measuring cup, combine the grated fresh ginger with the melted butter and pour this over the mangoes. Sprinkle ½ cup of the brown sugar over this and bake for 20 minutes, until the fruit is tender. Set aside.

3. Meanwhile, cream the soft butter and the remaining ¾ cup of brown sugar together in a large bowl. Add the vanilla, eggs, yogurt and semolina and mix thoroughly with a whisk. Add the candied ginger.

4. In a separate bowl, mix the flour, baking powder and cinnamon together. Gently mix the dry ingredients into the wet with a wooden spoon.

5. Drop this batter evenly over the mango in the pie plate. Bake for 30 minutes, until a knife comes out of the center clean. Allow it to cool completely before inverting onto a serving plate.

— *Moreka Jolar*

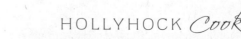

Peach-Berry Crisp with Cardamom

Pure warm fruit filling bubbles up through an oat-and-nut filled crumble topping bursting with fragrant cardamom. This recipe is versatile and forgiving and an easily be made without wheat and dairy and with variations on the fruit, nuts and seeds.

Preheat the oven to 350°F.

1. In a large bowl, combine the peaches and blueberries and gradually stir in the white flour. Set aside.

2. Using a food processor or blender, process the oats for 30 seconds or until they are coarsely ground.

3. In a large bowl, combine the ground oats with all the remaining dry ingredients. Mix the vanilla and maple syrup, if desired, into the melted butter and add to the dry mix. Combine until it is completely moist.

4. Pack the mixed fruit into the lightly oiled baking dish. Cover the fruit with the oat topping. Bake until the topping is brown and the fruit is tender. Serve hot from the oven or at room temperature.

VARIATIONS

A non-wheat flour can be substituted for the regular flour and the butter can be replaced with oil to create a wheat-free and dairy-free crisp. Add sunflower seeds, raisins or pumpkin seeds to the topping for a little variation. You can also add 1 tbsp fresh grated ginger to the fruit. Try other fruit combinations such as apple-blackberry, pear-raspberry or apricot-loganberry and omit the cardamom.

— *Moreka Jolar*

Serves 8-10

3 cups	sliced peaches	720 mL
2 cups	blueberries	480 mL
¼ cup	unbleached white flour	60 mL
1 cup	whole rolled oats	240 mL
½ cup	whole wheat flour	120 mL
½ cup	chopped nuts such as almonds or hazelnuts	120 mL
¼ cup	brown sugar or maple syrup	60 mL
1 tsp	cinnamon	5 mL
½ tsp	nutmeg	2.5 mL
½ tsp	ground cardamom	2.5 mL
¼ tsp	salt	1.2 mL
½ cup	melted butter	120 mL
1 tsp	vanilla extract	5 mL

*REQUIRES ONE **9**-INCH ROUND OR SQUARE BAKING DISH*

Pavlova

This is Australia's most famous contribution to the dessert world, created in honor
of the ballerina Anna Pavlova. These sweet meringues are cooked slowly and
at a low heat to give them a soft, chewy interior and a crispy outside.
Top them with whipped cream, sliced fruit and berries, and decorate them
generously with edible flower petals and you will have a
stunningly beautiful dessert.

Makes I dozen

I tsp	white wine vinegar	5 mL
I tsp	cornstarch	5 mL
I tsp	vanilla extract	5 mL
3	egg whites	3
¾ cup	white sugar	180 mL
I ½ cups	heavy cream	360 mL
½ lb.	fresh raspberries or sliced strawberries	230 g

Preheat the oven to 250°F.

1. In a small bowl, combine the vinegar, cornstarch and vanilla. Set aside.

2. In a large bowl, whip the egg whites until they form stiff peaks and then slowly add the sugar, mixing constantly.

3. Stir up the vinegar mixture and use a metal spoon to fold it into the egg whites.

4. Spoon this mixture into 12 equal portions onto parchment paper or a well-oiled baking sheet and bake for I ½ hours. Allow them to cool completely on cooling rack

5. Whip the cream for the topping. Top each pavlova with a dollop of whipped cream and fresh berries, garnish with a sprig of mint or lavender or with edible flower petals and serve immediately.

— *Chloe Gregg*

" The food at Hollyhock is absolutely
yummy and superb. There is so
much love in this food that you know when
you serve yourself that you will be more
healthy and happy from eating it. You
can feel it was prepared with care, with
love, and often that the salad, covered
with flowers, comes from the garden. It is
a feast for the eyes and for the taste buds.
And then to eat it outside facing such a
magnificent view, the ocean, the light
reflected on the waves is a treat for the
spirit that inspires awe, silence, convivi-
ality, conscious chewing and enjoyment
and gratitude for being here at this
wondrous place. "
— Margot Anand

Portuguese Rice Pudding

This is a traditional, creamy, slow-cooked rice pudding with a classic hint of lemon and cinnamon. Serve warm or at room temperature.

1. Use a sharp paring knife to cut the rind off the lemon in long strips, being careful to avoid as much of the white pith as possible.

2. In a heavy-bottomed saucepan, combine the milk, water, lemon rind, cinnamon stick and salt. Cover and bring to a boil. Stir in the rice, reduce heat to medium-low, and cook, uncovered for 30 to 40 minutes, until the rice is almost tender.

3. Add the sugar and continue cooking over low heat for 5 minutes, until the rice is completely tender and most of the liquid is absorbed. Remove from heat.

4. In a small bowl, beat the egg well and whisk it into the hot rice. Return the mixture to the heat and continue to stir until the pudding is slightly thickened, about 1 minute.

5. Remove the cinnamon stick and lemon rind, and then spoon the mixture into dessert dishes and sprinkle with ground cinnamon. Allow the pudding to cool and serve at room temperature.

— *Hanyu Wasyliw*

Serves 4-6

2 cups	milk	480 mL
2 cups	water	480 mL
1	lemon	1
1	cinnamon stick	1
¼ tsp	salt	1.2 mL
½ cup	short grain or arborio rice	120 mL
½ cup	white sugar	120 mL
1	egg	1
	ground cinnamon for garnish	

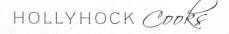

Power Cookies

Chocolate lovers will want to add a cup of dark chocolate chips to the dough of this energy-packed cookie, or press a chunk of dark or white chocolate into the center of each one before baking. The dough keeps in the refrigerator for up to a week or for a month in the freezer.
A vegan wonder.

Makes 1 dozen

1 cup	brown sugar	240 mL
1 cup	sunflower or safflower oil	240 mL
2 tsp	vanilla extract	10 mL
1 cup	whole wheat or spelt flour	240 mL
2 cups	whole rolled oats	480 mL
½ tsp	salt	2.5 mL
½ cup	pumpkin seeds	120 mL
½ cup	sesame seeds	120 mL
½ cup	flax seeds	120 mL
½ cup	sunflower seeds	120 mL

Preheat the oven to 350°F.

1. In a large bowl, cream the sugar with the oil and vanilla.

2. In a separate bowl, mix the flour, oats and salt until well combined.

3. Mix the dry ingredients well with the wet mixture. Add the seeds. This dough will be quite crumbly and will take a good deal of working with your hands to stick together.

4. Form the cookie dough into 12 firm patties and place them on a lightly oiled baking sheet. Bake for approximately 15-20 minutes, until the cookies are just turning brown. Allow the cookies to cool completely before lifting them off the sheet.

— *Ted Wallbridge*

cook's tip

Always toast your nuts and seeds. Whether they're for cookies, cakes, sauces or a main dish, toasting the nuts and seeds brings out their natural aroma and flavor. It's worth it.

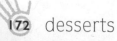
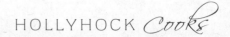

Sour Cream Cake

This is a basic, rich white cake for all occasions. Try out one of the variations below or get creative and try your own. Sprinkle the cooled cake with confectioners sugar or cocoa powder, top with your favorite frosting or whipped cream, fruit and edible flower blossoms such as roses.

Preheat the oven to 350°F.

1. In a large bowl, cream the butter and sugar together well. Mix in the 2 eggs, sour cream and vanilla.

2. In a separate bowl, combine the flour with the baking powder and baking soda. Combine the dry mixture into the wet and stir well.

3. Spoon batter into a lightly oil and floured Bundt pan. Bake for 50-60 minutes, until a toothpick comes out of the center clean. Allow the cake to cool 10 min. before inverting pan onto cooling rack. Allow the cake to cool completely before adding your desired topping or decoration.

VARIATIONS

• For a citrus-poppyseed cake, add ½ cup of poppyseeds and 1 tbsp of lemon zest to the batter.

• For a festive cake, add 1 cup of fresh cranberries and ¾ cup of chopped pecans.

• For chocolate swirl cake, mix ¼ cup cocoa with ⅓ cup sugar and lightly swirl this mixture into the batter.

— *Martha Abelson*

Serves 15-20

1 cup	soft butter	240 mL
1¼ cup	white sugar	300 mL
2	eggs	2
1 cup	sour cream	240 mL
1 tsp	vanilla extract	5 mL
2 cups	unbleached white flour	480 mL
2 tsp	baking powder	10 mL
½ tsp	baking soda	2.5 mL

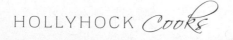

EIGHT

Breakfast

LET'S TAKE A MOMENT TO THINK ABOUT BREAKFAST. Let's sing its praises, consider what it does for us, what it does for others, what it could do for the world. Breakfast really does get the day off to the right start. Many of us feel like we're too busy to take the time to do more than shake something out of a mass-produced box, but when we settle into the idea of preparing and eating real food, there is a definite pay-off. We can think better, operate better, communicate better, and we feel better, when we have good food to fuel our bodies and minds. Our kids are easier to get along with when they have tasty and nutritious food in their stomachs. Getting along with a partner sure is easier when food takes the edge off morning crankiness. Yes, we'd all get along better if everyone took the time to sit down for a steaming hot bowl of oatmeal covered with stewed fruit, or baked eggs fresh out of the oven, or warm muffins with honey, or pancakes, or whatever food the morning called for.

The cooks at Hollyhock cooks have come up a myriad of simple, delicious and healthful ways to start every day with pleasure.

Applesauce Tahini Pudding

Served alone or over breakfast cereal, this thick, creamy mixture of apples and sesame
seed butter also works well as a dessert. It is naturally sweet or you can sweeten
it to taste with honey or maple syrup and, if it tickles your fancy, top it
with roasted nuts.

Serves 5

4 cups	thick and sweet applesauce	960 mL
1 cup	thick tahini	240 mL

1. Blend the applesauce and tahini in a blender, food processor or with a whisk until thoroughly combined. Chill for 1 hour before serving or make it a day in advance to leave extra time for chilling. The more you chill it, the thicker it will be. For a thicker consistency, increase the tahini.

— *Shivon Robinsong*

Baked Eggs

Baking eggs in a muffin tin makes them fit perfectly on top of an English muffin or bagel.
Combine some chopped fresh herbs to the eggs before baking. For Mexican baked
eggs, add one tablespoon of diced avocado and one tablespoon of
Pico De Gallo Salsa (page 97) to each egg after baking.

Serves 2

3	eggs	3
¼ cup	milk	60 mL
2 tbsp	freshly grated Swiss, sharp cheddar, chevre, or Gruyère cheese	30 mL
	dash of salt and pepper	

Preheat the oven to 400°F.

1. Whisk the eggs, milk, salt and pepper together and divide them evenly into 4 buttered muffin tins. Sprinkle the eggs with the grated cheese and bake at 400°F for 15 minutes or until the eggs puff up. Use a knife to slide around each egg to remove them from the pan.

— *Moreka Jolar*

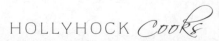
HOLLYHOCK *Cooks*

Black Rice Pudding with Banana and Lime

Nutty black Thai rice is combined in this recipe with creamy coconut milk, sweetened with banana, and given a hint of lime to create this rich, purple-colored breakfast sensation. It's a sweet way to say good morning to anyone.

1. In a small, covered saucepan, bring the rice and water to a boil. Reduce the heat and allow the rice to simmer for 20 minutes.

2. Add the coconut milk, banana and lime zest, cover the pan again, and allow the mixture to simmer on very low for 30 minutes. Serve hot, garnished with toasted coconut.

* Look for black Thai rice in Asian food stores.

— *Moreka Jolar*

2 servings

½ cup	black Thai rice *	120 mL
1 cup	water	240 mL
¾ cup	coconut milk	180 mL
1	banana finely diced	1
½ tsp	lime zest	2.5 mL
	toasted coconut to garnish	

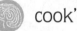 **cook's tip**

Coconut toasts very quickly. It is best to toast it in a small frying pan on low heat.

Breakfast Corn Soufflé

This is a hearty cornmeal soufflé packed with vegetable flavor and your favorite cheese. It is so hearty that it will not fall like more fragile soufflés. Serve with Pico De Gallo Salsa (page 97) or Baked Beans (page 82). Add chili or cayenne for a little more heat. It's a good choice for Sunday brunch.

Serves 8-10

2 tbsp	sunflower or safflower oil	30 mL
I cup	finely diced red bell peppers	240 mL
½ cup	finely diced onions	120 mL
½ cup	finely diced carrots	120 mL
I cup	corn kernels, fresh off the cob or frozen	240 mL
½ tsp	minced garlic	2.5 mL
I tsp	black pepper	5 mL
2 cups	water	480 mL
½ tsp	salt	2.5 mL
½ cup	yellow cornmeal	120 mL
2	eggs	2
I cup	milk or dairy alternative	240 mL
1½ cups	your favorite grated cheese	360 mL
¼ cup	chopped fresh parsley	60 mL

REQUIRES A 9x13-INCH BAKING DISH

Preheat the oven to 350°F.

1. In a small frying pan, sauté the bell peppers, onions, carrots, corn, garlic and black pepper in the oil until the carrots are tender. Set this aside.

2. In a saucepan, bring the water and salt to a boil and slowly pour in the cornmeal, whisking vigorously. Immediately remove from the heat and continue to whisk until thickened.

3. In a small bowl, whisk together the eggs and milk and then mix them slowly into the cornmeal. Add the sautéed vegetables, stir well and then add the grated cheese and parsley. Transfer to the lightly oiled, 9x13-inch baking dish and bake at 350°F for 45 minutes to I hour, or until it sets.

— *Moreka Jolar*

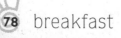
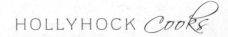
HOLLYHOCK *Cooks*

Hummus with Roasted
Red Peppers (top) page 110

White Bean Spread
with Roasted Garlic
and Sage page 112

Lemon Squares page 167

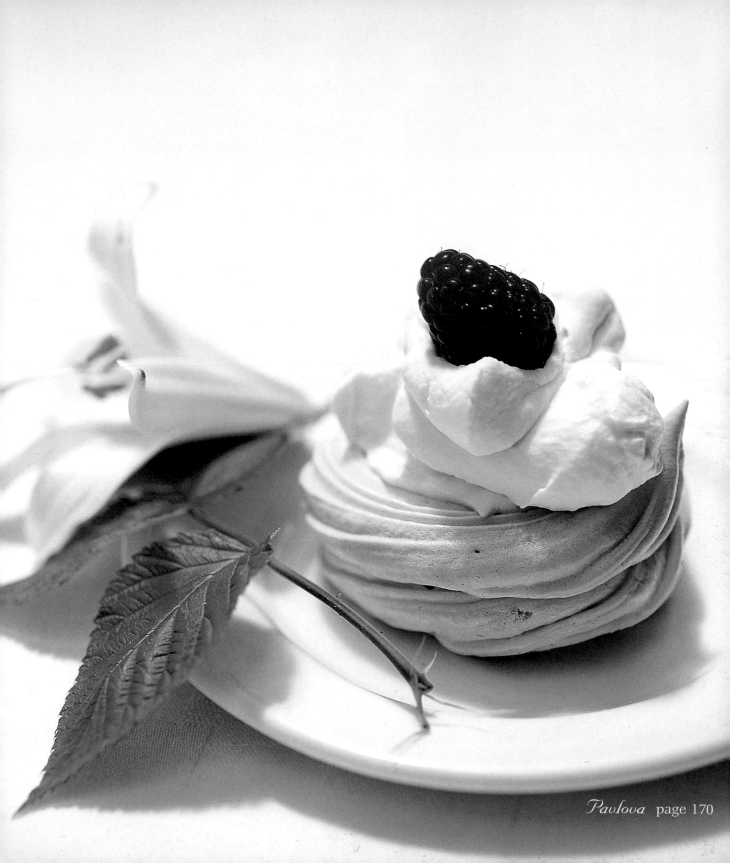

Pavlova page 170

Hollyhock Granola page 184,
Soy Yogurt and Dreamy
Whole Wheat Scones page 128

Breakfast Custard with Fresh Apricots

Good old comfort food, this light and silky custard is healthy, too. The apricots provide the perfect soft and tart addition. This custard is baked in a *bain-marie* or water bath to minimize curdling, so be sure to use a baking dish that will fit comfortably into another.

Preheat the oven to 350°F.

1. In a blender, mix the eggs and vanilla until foamy.

2. Cut the apricots in half, discarding the pits, and arrange them open-side down in the bottom of a buttered, 8x10-inch glass baking dish.

3. In a saucepan, scald the milk, being careful not to boil it. When the milk is steaming hot, stir in the honey and remove it from the heat. Slowly add the egg mixture to the hot milk, stirring constantly. Pour this on top of the apricots in the baking dish. Sprinkle with nutmeg. Set this dish into another larger baking dish and fill this one with 1 inch of boiling water. Bake at 350° F for 30 minutes, or just until a knife comes out of the center clean. Allow it to cool and then set for 15 minutes. Serve warm or chilled.

— *Moreka Jolar*

Serves 6-8

5	ripe apricots	5
3 cups	milk, or dairy substitute	720 mL
¼ cup	honey	60 mL
4	eggs	4
2 tsp	vanilla	10 mL
	a sprinkle of nutmeg	

REQUIRES AN 8x10-INCH GLASS BAKING DISH

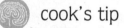 **cook's tip**

Avoid baking custards and soufflés in convection ovens. They do not like the vibration of the fan. A traditional gas or electric oven works best.

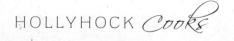 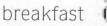

Breakfast Oatmeal Two Ways

Here are two great ways to make oatmeal even more wonderful. The first gives quantities for the perfect bowl of tender, cooked oats. The second involves toasting the oats prior to cooking them. Toasting the oats before boiling them makes a flaky and nutty-flavored cereal and is worth the extra time.

Serves 2

BASIC OATS

2 cups	water	480 mL
1½ cups	whole rolled oats	360 mL

TOASTY OATS

2 cups	water	480 mL
1½ cups	whole rolled oats	360 mL

BASIC OATS

1. Bring the water to a boil and add the oats. Cover the pot and reduce the heat to low. Allow it to simmer for approximately 5 minutes on low heat. Stir frequently to keep the oatmeal from sticking. Remove the lid and simmer if you would like a drier oatmeal. Cook until the oatmeal reaches the consistency you like.

TOASTY OATS

1. In a saucepan, dry-toast the oats on medium heat. Stir often and toast them until the oats are browning. This should take about 10 minutes. Add boiling water, cover and simmer on low heat for approximately 5 minutes. Stir occasionally. If you like a drier, denser oatmeal, remove the cover to allow more water to evaporate.

VARIATIONS

To either oatmeal, add a pinch of cinnamon, nutmeg, or cardamom, a handful of chopped almonds, hazelnuts, coconut, sunflower seeds, flax seeds, pumpkin seeds, or soy nuts while your oats are cooking. Or toast the nuts first if you prefer the toasted flavor. Dice up an apple, pear, banana, dried apricots, prunes, cherries or blueberries and cook. Top with brown sugar, maple syrup, honey or milk, stir in some protein powder, or add some granola for crunch.

— *Moreka Jolar*

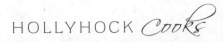

Cardamom Yogurt Sauce

This sweet, creamy sauce is infused with the warming taste of cardamom and the fresh tang of citrus. Serve over pancakes or fresh fruit salad, or even as a dip with sliced fruits.

1. In a small bowl, whisk all the ingredients together and refrigerate for at least 1 hour.

— *Hanyu Wasyliw*

Serves 4-6

1 cup	yogurt	240 mL
1 tbsp	white sugar	15 mL
2 tbsp	orange juice concentrate	30 mL
1 tsp	lime zest	5 mL
¼ tsp	ground cardamom	1.2 mL
	a dash of salt	

Cornmeal Buttermilk Pancakes

These fluffy pancakes have the flavor of zesty buttermilk and the light crunch of cornmeal. Serve them topped with fresh fruit and yogurt for a perfect breakfast.

1. In a large bowl, combine all the dry ingredients.
2. In a small bowl, beat the two egg whites until they form stiff peaks. Set aside.
3. In a third bowl, mix the buttermilk, melted butter or oil, the 2 beaten eggs and lemon zest. Combine the wet ingredients with the dry and mix thoroughly. Fold in the beaten egg whites. Cook in a medium-hot, lightly oiled skillet or griddle.

— *Moreka Jolar*

Serves 6-8

½ cup	whole wheat flour	120 mL
½ cup	unbleached white flour	120 mL
½ cup	cornmeal	120 mL
¼ cup	brown sugar	60 mL
1¼ tsp	baking powder	6.25 mL
¼ tsp	baking soda	1.2 mL
¼ tsp	salt	1.2 mL
2	egg whites	2
1¼ cup	buttermilk	300 mL
2	eggs beaten	2
4 tbsp	melted butter or sunflower oil	60 mL
1 tbsp	lemon zest	15 mL

Easy Whole Wheat Crêpes

Here is a light and nutritious way to start your day. These whole wheat crêpes can be stuffed with sweet fruit and berries or savory grilled vegetables. The batter will keep well in a sealed container refrigerated for up to five days.

Serves 4-6

½ cup	whole wheat or spelt flour	120 mL
½ cup	milk or soy milk	120 mL
¼ cup	water	60 mL
2	eggs	2
2 tbsp	melted butter	30 mL
1½ tbsp	sugar	23 mL
	pinch of salt	

 cook's tip

Recipes made with soy milk tend to stick to the pan more than cow's milk. Always be sure to generously oil pans to avoid this nasty sticking.

1. In a blender, mix all the ingredients on high speed until smooth. Let the blended mixture sit for 20-30 minutes for the best results.

2. Heat a non-stick skillet on low heat. If you used soy milk instead of milk, oil the pan slightly before cooking each crêpe. Pour just enough batter in to swirl around and evenly cover the bottom of the skillet. Cook the crêpe until it begins to bubble and then flip and brown both sides. Keep each crêpe covered with a tea towel and warm in an oven at 200°F until serving.

3. Fill with fresh fruit and berries and, if you like, add regular or soy yogurt and then roll it carefully up. Top with maple syrup.

— *Sylvie Rousseau*

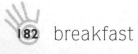

 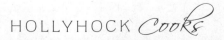

Hearty No-Wheat Pancakes

This forgiving recipe allows you to experiment with different types of flour to suit special diets or tastes. This yields the most hearty and filling pancakes you will ever stumble across. The recipe can also be altered to suit a vegan diet.

1. In a large bowl, combine all the dry ingredients.

2. In a separate bowl, mix the milk, yogurt, oil, eggs and vanilla well. Add the wet mixture to the dry ingredients, stirring with a fork until blended, but be careful not to over-mix. Add the fruit if desired. The oat flour will thicken as the batter stands so it may be necessary to add more milk until the batter is just pourable.

3. Cook in a preheated and lightly oiled cast-iron skillet on medium heat. Flip when the pancake starts to bubble. Serve with any of the following: butter, fruit, yogurt, jam, molasses, syrup, whipped cream or strawberries.

VARIATIONS

A vegan version of this recipe can be made if you add more sticky rice flour and eliminate the yogurt and eggs. Use two teaspoons of lemon juice to help this mixture rise.

— *David Rousseau*

Makes 10 large pancakes

2 cups	rolled oats ground into flour in blender	480 mL
1 cup	barley flour, spelt, amaranth or buckwheat	240 mL
1 cup	sticky rice flour or rice gluten	240 mL
½ cup	soy protein powder, if desired	120 mL
3 tbsp	brown sugar	45 mL
1 tsp	baking powder	5 mL
½ tsp	baking soda	2.5 mL
½ tsp	salt	2.5 mL
2 cups	milk or dairy substitute	480 mL
¾ cup	yogurt	180 mL
½ cup	sunflower or safflower oil	120 mL
2	eggs beaten	2
½ tsp	vanilla	2.5 mL
1 cup	fresh or partially thawed berries or sliced bananas, if desired	240 mL

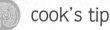 cook's tip

Here is an easy and delicious non-dairy alternative to whipped cream. Whisk or beat canned coconut cream, add sugar if you like, cover and refrigerate overnight and you will have a thick and decadent spreadable cream.

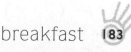

Hollyhock Granola

For as long as we can remember, a generous bowl heaped with this granola has graced
every breakfast buffet table at Hollyhock. Packed with toasty oat and seed flavor,
it is nutritious and filling. After the granola is cool, a nice variation is to add
two cups of raisins, dried blueberries, cranberries, chopped dry apricots,
or toasted cashews. The granola will keep well
for one month in a sealed container.

Makes about 10 cups

6 cups	whole rolled oats	1.4 L
1 cup	sunflower seeds	240 mL
1 cup	unsweetened shredded coconut	240 mL
½ cup	pumpkin seeds	120 mL
¼ cup	unhulled sesame seeds	60 mL
2 tsp	cinnamon	10 mL
⅔ cup	sunflower or safflower oil	160 mL
⅔ cup	honey	160 mL
2 tsp	vanilla	10 mL

Preheat the oven to 250°F.

1. In a large bowl, combine all the dry ingredients.

2. In a saucepan, heat the oil and the honey at low heat until the honey melts. Don't allow the honey and oil to boil. Take the honey and oil off the stove and add the vanilla. Pour this mixture over the dry ingredients and toss them well until the granola is shiny and well coated.

3. Spread the mixture onto 2 baking sheets and bake until golden, stirring every 20 minutes. It takes about an hour to bake at 250°F and less time at a higher heat. The granola may still be slightly soft when it comes out of the oven but it will crisp up as it cools. Cool completely before storing in an airtight container.

* Instead of sesame seeds you can use 1 cup (240 mL) of slivered or chopped almonds or ¼ cup (60 mL) of flax seeds.

— *Joy Shipway*

" The food at Hollyhock has a special
quality of harmony and tenderness
in it. In eating it, I always feel I am
being fed directly by both the male and
female energies of the landscape of
Cortes Island and of British
Columbia, and so I am being at once
energized and calmed."
— Andrew Harvey

Lavender Fruit Salad

Ripe tropical fruits and strawberries are combined in this recipe with fresh, fragrant lavender blossoms to make this fruit salad an exotic taste sensation.
Top it with yogurt and a sprinkle of granola.

1. In a small bowl, combine all the fruits and lavender blossoms and serve immediately.

— Moreka Jolar

Serves 2

1 cup	cubed mango	240 mL
1 cup	thinly sliced strawberries	240 mL
3	kiwi fruits peeled and sliced in rounds	3
1 tsp	fresh lavender flowers	5 mL

Maple Brown Rice Pudding

This hot rice cereal is infused with the classic rice pudding flavors of cinnamon and lemon, and is naturally sweetened with maple syrup. It's a toasty way to start your day and is an excellent way to use up leftover brown rice.

1. In a small saucepan, bring the cooked rice, the milk, cinnamon stick and lemon zest to a simmer. Cover and simmer gently for 45 minutes. Stir every 10 minutes or use a heat diffuser so it doesn't stick and burn. Add the maple syrup and serve.

— Moreka Jolar

Serves 2

2 cups	cooked brown rice, short grain is best	480 mL
1 cup	milk or dairy alternative	240 mL
½	cinnamon stick	½
½ tsp	lemon zest	2.5 mL
1 tbsp	maple syrup	15 mL

Melon and Berry Salad

This intriguing fruit salad uses a half melon as its bowl. It is exquisite to look at, delicious to taste, and it leaves nothing to waste. Any other fruit such as kiwis, oranges, apples, bananas and mangoes can be used in place of the berries.

6-8 servings

½	ripe honeydew or cantaloupe melon	½
3 cups	ripe large berries such as blackberries, loganberries or raspberries	720 mL

1. Cut the melon in half. To help the half melon sit straight when full of salad, take a thin slice of the skin off the bottom to make a flat surface to anchor the bowl. Discard the melon seeds and using a melon baller or small ice cream scoop, scoop out the melon. Combine the melon balls with the berries and place them back into the melon bowl. Mix the salad with rose petals or sunflower petals to make it even more beautiful.

— *Moreka Jolar*

Muesli with Dried Cranberries and Coconut

Muesli is a classic European breakfast cereal made with oats, dried fruit and nuts, grated apple and yogurt. This filling and nutritious cereal is made on the previous night and refrigerated to allow the raw oats to absorb all the moisture. Soy yogurt works very well as a non-dairy substitute and you can also experiment with different nuts, seeds or other dried fruits or berries.

Serves 5-6

1 cup	whole rolled oats	240 mL
½ cup	dry unsweetened cranberries	120 mL
⅓ cup	toasted slivered almonds	80 mL
⅓ cup	unsweetened shredded coconut	80 mL
¼ cup	thinly sliced dry apricots	60 mL
1 tsp	cinnamon	5 mL
	pinch of nutmeg	
2 cups	yogurt	480 mL
1 cup	shredded apple	240 mL

1. In a large bowl, combine all of the dry ingredients well before mixing in the yogurt and apple. Refrigerate overnight and enjoy the next morning. Add more yogurt each day if you want to keep it really moist. The oats will continue to soak up all the moisture.

— *Moreka Jolar*

HOLLYHOCK *Cooks*

Oven-Baked Yam and Potato Hash

Yams are a sweet, warm ingredient in hash browns. The process of baking these slightly sweet hashbrowns yields a less oily but still crunchy breakfast sensation. They are fast and easy to prepare. Serve them hot with Baked Eggs (page 176) or Scrambled Tofu (page 187), and, if you like, sprinkle them with a little shredded Parmesan while baking.

Preheat the oven to 450°F.

1. Mix the yams, potatoes, onions and garlic well and coat thoroughly with oil and salt. Spread in a thin layer on 2 lightly oiled baking sheets and bake at 450°F until the top begins to brown and crisp. This will take approximately 30 minutes. Using a spatula, turn the hash over and bake for another 30 minutes until the other side has browned. Serve hot.

— *Moreka Jolar*

Serves 4-6

8 cups	grated unpeeled yams	1.9 L
8 cups	grated unpeeled potatoes	1.9 L
3 cups	grated onions	720 mL
1 tbsp	minced garlic	15 mL
¼ cup	sunflower or safflower oil	60 mL
1 tsp	salt	5 mL

Scrambled Tofu

Scrambled tofu is a protein-packed alternative to eggs in the morning. Full of fresh vegetable flavor with a light curry taste, have a balanced start to your day with this savory, low-fat scramble.

1. In a large skillet, sauté all the ingredients, except the parsley and scallions, until the vegetables are tender and the water from the tofu has evaporated, about 20 minutes. Remove from the heat and toss in the parsley and scallions. Serve.

— *Moreka Jolar*

Serves 6

1 lb.	soft crumbled tofu	460 g
2 cups	sliced mushrooms	480 mL
1 cup	diced onions	240 mL
1 cup	diced celery	240 mL
1 cup	diced bell peppers	240 mL
1 cup	thinly sliced zucchini	240 mL
2 tsp	crushed garlic	10 mL
2 tsp	vegetable salt such as Spike or Herbamere	10 mL
1½ tsp	turmeric	7.5 mL
1 tsp	curry powder	5 mL
1 tsp	black pepper	5 mL
¼ cup	chopped fresh parsley	60 mL
¼ cup	diced chives or scallions	60 mL

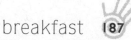

Soy Hotcakes with Orange

This pancake recipe incorporates soy flour into the ingredients, keeping it lower in carbohydrates and high in protein. There is just a hint of orange.

Makes 10-12 small cakes

I cup	whole wheat, spelt or teff flour	240 mL
⅓ cup	soy flour	80 mL
I tsp	baking powder	5 mL
½ tsp	baking soda	2.5 mL
	pinch of salt	
2	eggs, separated	2
2 cups	milk or dairy substitute	480 mL
2 tbsp	sunflower or safflower oil	30 mL
I tsp	orange zest	5 mL

1. In a medium-sized bowl, combine all of the dry ingredients.

2. Separate the eggs and combine the yolks with milk, oil, and zest in a second bowl.

3. In a third bowl, whip the egg whites until they form soft peaks.

4. Add the milk mixture to the dry mixture and stir it gently. Fold in the egg whites. Pour approximately ½ cup of batter into a lightly oiled and preheated cast-iron skillet or griddle. Cook both sides until golden. Keep warm in the oven until serving.

— *Moreka Jolar*

cook's tip

Pancakes are ready to flip when small bubbles appear on top.

Soy Yogurt

Soy yogurt is easy to make, nutritious and an excellent non-dairy alternative to yogurt. It is silky and thick and packed with protein. Add fruit compote or berries to heighten the delight of it.

Makes 2 cups

12 oz.	firm silken-style tofu	340 g
½ cup	orange juice concentrate	120 mL
½ tsp	vanilla extract	120 mL
I tbsp	honey, barley malt, rice syrup or maple syrup, if desired	15 mL
¼ tsp	nutmeg, if desired	2.5 mL

1. Mix all the ingredients in a food processor or blender until they are extremely smooth. This should take about 2 minutes. Serve with your breakfast cereal or even as a light dessert.

— *Moreka Jolar*

Stewed Fruit

Our stewed fruit recipe turns an ordinary bowl of oatmeal into sweet and nutrient-rich gourmet breakfast event. It stores well in the refrigerator and can be easily reheated.

1. In a heavy saucepan, place all the ingredients and add enough water to just cover the fruit. Bring to a boil and reduce heat to a low simmer for approximately 25 minutes, until everything is tender and soupy. Serve hot over morning oatmeal or with yogurt.

VARIATIONS
Add a couple of inches of sliced ginger and ½ cup chopped figs, if desired.

— Moreka Jolar

Makes 5 cups

I cup	whole pitted prunes	240 mL
I cup	whole dried apricots	240 mL
½ cup	raisins	120 mL
½ cup	chopped dry dates	120 mL
I	chopped apple	I
I	peeled and chopped orange	I
I	chopped banana	I
I	cinnamon stick	I

Sweet Oat Bake with Currants

Tired of standard oatmeal? Try this. Eggs and milk and honey are combined with oats and currants and baked into a sweet and hearty custard with a trace of nutmeg.

Preheat the oven to 350°F.

1. In a blender, combine the milk, eggs, water, honey and vanilla until foamy. Pour this into a lightly buttered 9-inch-square baking pan. Add the oats and stir gently. Top with the currants and sprinkle with nutmeg. Bake for 20-25 minutes until firm. Serve it warm, topped with yogurt and fruit.

— Moreka Jolar

Serves 5-6

I cup	milk or dairy alternative	240 mL
2	eggs	2
½ cup	water	120 mL
2 tbsp	honey	30 mL
½ tsp	vanilla	2.5 mL
I cup	whole rolled oats	240 mL
¼ cup	currants	60 mL
	nutmeg to sprinkle on top	

REQUIRES ONE 9-INCH SQUARE BAKING DISH

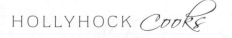 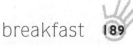

Toasted Multigrain and Seed Cereal

This recipe gives instructions for making your own hot multigrain cereal mix. The grains, nuts and seeds are toasted to bring out their natural robust tastes and then ground in a food processor. This mixture will keep when in a sealed jar for up to one month and you can follow the instructions below to cook it. The almonds and quinoa make this cereal high in protein and calcium, and the pumpkin seeds are rich in iron.

Makes 4 cups dry

½ cup	whole almonds	120 mL
½ cup	whole pumpkin seeds	120 mL
½ cup	quinoa	120 mL
½ cup	millet	120 mL
½ cup	brown rice	120 mL
¼ cup	unhulled sesame seeds	60 mL
¼ cup	flax seeds	60 mL

1. In a large cast-iron skillet, toast the almonds and pumpkin seeds until the seeds begin to brown and pop. Add the remaining whole grains and seeds and continue to toast for another 15 minutes. They should all snap and pop. Continue to stir.

2. Remove from the heat and allow the mixture to cool completely before mixing in a food processor for 20 seconds or so. It's nice to keep some of the grainy texture, so don't mix it for too long. This is the base to make your own hot multigrain cereal. It will keep in a sealed jar in a cool dry spot for up to 1 month. Any longer and it should be kept in the refrigerator or freezer.

TO COOK THE CEREAL

1. In a small saucepan, bring 2 cups of water to a boil. Add 1 cup of the dry cereal, cover and reduce to a simmer for 20 minutes. Stir occasionally. Serve hot.

— *Moreka Jolar*

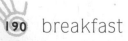

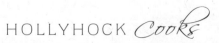

NINE

Drinks

THE INSPIRATION FOR MANY OF THE DRINKS at Hollyhock comes, once again, from the garden. Fresh herbs and flowers make delicious, refreshing teas. Berries and fresh fruit are perfect for smoothies. On cold rainy days, Mexican Hot Chocolate, Chai, or Hot Apple Cider warm you up.

One of the most beautiful sights of the summer is the small basket of fresh tea herbs on the drinks table in the main lodge. This basket is filled with sprigs of herbs and petals of flowers, according to the season. Lemon balm, raspberry leaf, bee balm, hyssop, lavender, rose petals and chamomile flowers are offered in a fragrant arrangement. Infusions of mixtures of these delicate herbs yield scents and flavors that commercially grown teas can't match.

Another staple at the drink table are the two pitchers of cold tea: the mellow Hollyhock Kitsilano Tea and the spicy Hollyhock Ginger Tea. There is nothing like these teas, drunk separately, or mixed together, to cool you off on a hot day.

Remember to drink plenty of water every day and also be sure to indulge in our luxurious alternatives to the basic life brew.

Banana-Berry Smoothie

On Cortes Island we have an abundance of blackberries in the summer. Heaps of them go into making smoothies like these. What an exquisite way to start the day.

Serves 2

1½ cups	fresh orange juice or the juice of 4 oranges	360 mL
1 cup	frozen berries such as blueberries, strawberries, blackberries or raspberries	240 mL
1	peeled banana	1

1. Combine all ingredients in a blender and mix until smooth. Serve immediately.

— Moreka Jolar

Chai

Chai is a sweet, spiced and aromatic Indian tea that is bold in taste. Double this recipe and drink it all day. The cardamom seeds neutralize the effect of the caffeine in the black tea, giving it a gentle uplifting quality that won't fry your nerves.

Makes 6 cups

9 cups	water	2.2 L
¼ cup	freshly grated ginger	60 mL
2	large cinnamon sticks	2
2 tsp	whole cardamom seeds	10 mL
12	whole cloves	12
2	whole star anise or 2 tsp whole fennel seeds	2
2	black tea bags, a good Indian tea is best	2
3 cups	milk or non-dairy alternative	720 mL
1 tsp	vanilla	5 mL
	sweetener as desired	

1. In a large saucepan, boil the water with the ginger, cinnamon, cardamom, cloves and star anise or fennel until only ⅓ of its original volume is remaining, about 3 cups. Remove from the heat, add the tea bags, cover and allow to steep for 10 minutes.

2. Put this through a sieve to strain off the whole spices and tea bags and gently reheat with the milk and vanilla extract added. Sweeten to taste and serve hot or chilled.

— Moreka Jolar

Coconut Mango Smoothie

This is a wonderful, thick and naturally sweet smoothie that is great for breakfast. Throw in a scoop of protein powder and it'll keep you going all day long. Serve it topped with a sprinkle of toasted coconut. For a refreshing and icy drink, freeze the fruit beforehand.

1. Peel and cut the mango flesh off the pit. Blend all the ingredients together in a blender. Serve immediately.

— *Moreka Jolar*

Serves 2

1	ripe mango	1
½ cup	pitted cherries	120 mL
½ cup	yogurt or soy yogurt	120 mL
1 cup	milk, non-dairy alternative or juice	240 mL
¼ cup	shredded coconut	60 mL

Fairy Tea

Imagine what fairies would drink. Hot water infused with spearmint and chamomile and lavender flowers would help a fairy lift her wings. Combine the fresh herbs and blossoms in large portions, lay out in a basket to dry in the sun and place in a sealed jar to give as an elegant gift. If these ingredients are not available to you fresh, dried spearmint and flowers will also be fine for the tea.

1. Combine all of the ingredients and place 3 tbsp of this fresh tea in a large teapot, cover with boiling water and allow it 5 minutes to steep. Try adding some of your favorite juice to this tea and drink it chilled.

* In order to capture the natural fragrant oils of the lavender in foods, it's best to harvest it right before the buds open.

— *Moreka Jolar*

2 parts	fresh spearmint leaves
1 part	fresh rose petals
1 part	fresh young lavender flowers *
1 part	fresh chamomile flowers

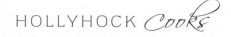

Hollyhock Ginger Tea

Ginger's refreshing and cleansing properties make this tea a wonderful drink on a hot day. Heated, it is an immune-system builder when you feel a cold coming on. This tea is by far the drink of choice at Hollyhock.

Makes 6 cups

8 cups	water	1.9 L
½ cup	diced fresh ginger	120 mL
⅓ cup	honey	80 mL
½ cup	fresh lemon juice	120 mL

1. Boil the ginger in 4 cups of the water for 20 minutes. Remove from heat and dissolve the honey into the brew. Strain off the ginger, and then transfer the liquid to a jug. Add the lemon juice and the remaining 4 cups of water. Serve it warm or chilled.

Hollyhock Kitsilano Tea

This iced tea is rich in vitamin C and brilliant pink in color, due to the hibiscus flowers. Serve it on its own or combined with fruit juice or Hollyhock Ginger Tea.

Makes 6 cups

6 cups	water	1.4 L
⅓ cup	dried chamomile	80 mL
½ cup	dried hibiscus flowers	120 mL
½ cup	dried peppermint	120 mL
⅓ cup	honey	80 mL

1. Bring 4 cups of the water to a boil and pour it over all the herbs and the honey. Cover and allow the tea to steep for 15 minutes. Place a piece of cheesecloth or a coffee filter in a strainer and strain the herbs from the tea. Add the remaining 2 cups of cold water and serve it chilled.

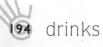

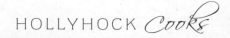
HOLLYHOCK *Cooks*

Hot Apple Cider

A crisp fall day calls for a cup of steaming hot apple cider and a romp in the leaves. This warming cider is made with hot apple juice infused with the irresistible and aromatic flavors of cinnamon, allspice, cloves and orange.

1. Use a paring knife and carefully cut the peel off the orange, getting as little pith or white of the skin as possible.

2. Heat all the ingredients in a saucepan and allow it to simmer for up to 1 hour. Serve it hot.

VARIATIONS

To spice things up, add a couple of slices of fresh ginger while the cider cooks. Or use 1 part apple cider with 1 part cranberry to create a more tart taste.

— *Moreka Jolar*

Makes 6 cups

6 cups	unfiltered apple juice	1.4 L
1	cinnamon stick	1
6	whole allspice berries	6
4	whole cloves	4
	peel of 1 orange	

cook's tip

When using the skin of citrus fruit always use organic fruit. Non-organic citrus fruits contain high concentrations of pesticides. If you can't find organic be sure to wash the fruit well with hot, soapy water.

Mexican Hot Chocolate

This rich hot chocolate is spiced with the traditional Mexican tastes of cinnamon, chili and vanilla. The chili spice is mild but is just enough to warm you to your toes. This is also easy to prepare without dairy, by using an alternative such as soy milk.

1. In a small bowl, combine the cocoa powder, sugar, cinnamon and chili. Add the water and vanilla. Whisk this into a paste.

2. Heat the milk or non-dairy alternative in a saucepan. Be careful not to let it boil. When it is hot, whisk the chocolate mix into it. Serve it hot.

— *Moreka Jolar*

Makes 6 cups

½ cup	cocoa powder	120 mL
¼ cup	brown sugar	60 mL
1 tsp	cinnamon	5 mL
½ tsp	chili powder	2.5 mL
½ cup	water	120 mL
1 tsp	vanilla	5 mL
5 cups	milk or non-dairy alternative	1.2 L

Peaches and Cream

When the peaches ripen to perfection, blend them with coconut milk into a divine nectar.
Double the quantities and fill up the popsicle trays for a treat kids of all ages will enjoy.

Serves 2

2	ripe peaches	2
I cup	sliced strawberries	240 mL
I	frozen banana	I
½ cup	coconut milk	120 mL

1. Cut the peaches off the pit and blend them with the remaining ingredients in a blender or food processor.

— *Moreka Jolar*

Tiger's Milk

Tiger's milk is a form of eggnog with a healthy dose of iron from the molasses and vitamin B from the nutritional flake yeast. It is a very healthy way to go completely nutritious first thing in the morning. Tiger's milk will keep for two days when refrigerated.

Serves 2

2 cups	milk or non-dairy alternative	480 mL
I	egg, if desired	I
2 tbsp	molasses	30 mL
I tbsp	nutritional flake yeast	15 mL
½ tsp	vanilla	2.5 mL

1. Combine all the ingredients in a blender. Serve immediately.

— *David Rousseau*

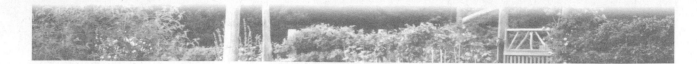

HOLLYHOCK OFFERS GUESTS THREE FULL MEALS DAILY, complete with freshly baked breads, pastries and a host of original dishes and desserts. We have a staff who prepare, cook, serve, and clean up every day, enabling us to turn out gourmet food for large numbers of people, while enjoying what we're doing. You probably can't do what we do at home, but what you can do is take a cue from us and rely on the freshest ingredients possible and your own creativity.

The following selection of a week of Hollyhock menus is meant to offer you inspiration and ideas for all occasions. These menus can be used for planning a dinner party for a large number of people or for getting some great new ideas for cooking at home for yourself, your family or friends. With food that is local and fresh, the spirit of Hollyhock's cooking can be replicated in any kitchen.

A Week at the Hollyhock Table

Day 1

BREAKFAST
Hollyhock Granola

Baked Eggs

Zucchini Bread

Lavender Fruit Salad with yogurt

LUNCH
Spicy Squash Soup with Roasted Garlic and Yogurt

Spinach Feta Rolls

Green Bean and Smoked Salmon Salad

green salad

MIDDLE EASTERN DINNER
Spanakopita with Green Olives and Artichoke Hearts

Green Bean Greek Salad

Hummus with Roasted Red Peppers

Tzatziki

Pita Bread with Sesame Seeds

Roasted Roots with Lemon and Rosemary

Layered Nut Torte

Day 2 BREAKFAST
Toasty Oats
Scrambled Tofu
Melon and Berry Salad
Fruit Turnovers with Ginger and Cardamom

LUNCH
Filo Bake with Leeks and Shitake Mushrooms
Yellow Beans with Honey Balsamic Vinaigrette and Oven-Roasted Tomatoes
Spinach Salad with Toasted Seeds
Chocolate Oatmeal Cookies with Orange

MEDITERRANEAN DINNER
Roasted Vegetable Lasagne
Antipasto Platter
Roasted Garlic Focaccia with Dry Black Olives
bowls of olive oil and balsamic vinegar for dipping
Arugula, Pear and Romano Salad
Lemon Squares

Day 3 BREAKFAST
Soy Hotcakes with Orange
Cardamom Yogurt Sauce
Stewed Fruit
Soft Boiled Free-Range Eggs
Hot Apple Cider

LUNCH
Black Bean Soup with Chipotle and Orange
sour cream and Mango Salsa to garnish
Best Ever Cornbread
veggie sticks with Caesar Tofu Dip
green salad

WEST COAST BARBECUE DINNER

Barbecued Salmon with Mixed Garden Herbs

Roasted Barley Pilaf with Mushrooms and Hazelnuts

Granary Buns

Bell Peppers Stuffed with Cherry Tomatoes

green salad

Cream Puffs filled with whipped cream and berries

BREAKFAST

Hearty No-Wheat Pancakes with

Honey Rose Butter and

Applesauce Tahini Pudding

Baked Eggs with salsa and sharp cheddar

LUNCH

Dal

Baked Samosas with

Banana Chutney

Green Beans Indian Style

green salad

Power Cookies

ASIAN DINNER

Thai Peanut Tofu with

Thai Red Curry Sauce

Black Thai Rice with chopped mango to garnish

jasmine rice

Pickled Arame Salad

Carrot and Asparagus Sesame Stir-fry

Won Ton Chips

Banana-Berry Ice

Day 5   BREAKFAST

Breakfast Corn Soufflé

Sesame Home Fries

Banana-Berry Smoothie

LUNCH

Prawn and Snapper Stew with Leeks and White Wine

Fennel-Topped French Bread with Garlic-Rosemary Butter

Spinach Salad with Crispy Apple and Toasted Cashews

EAST INDIAN DINNER

Vegetable Korma

Fragrant Saffron Rice

Sweet Potato and Chard Curry

Coconut Cilantro Chutney

Green Apple Raita

Baked Pappadums

Mango Ginger Upside-Down Cake

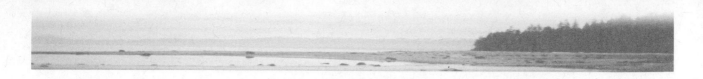

COOKING FOR LARGE NUMBERS of people can be intimidating, exhilarating and one of life's greatest ways to nurture a lot of people at the same time. Hollyhock has twenty years of experience in this genre of meal preparation. Here are a few tricks we've picked up along the way to make cooking for large numbers a success.

How to Cook Successfully for Large Numbers of People

1. TAKE A MOMENT TO VISUALIZE THE MEAL. Visualize the complete array of colors, tastes and textures.

2. CHECK YOUR SERVING PLATTERS. Make sure you have the utensils and dishes to realize your vision.

3. GAUGE YOUR ENERGY. From that, plan the menu. If you have a lot of energy and can't wait to dig your hands into something creative, you can choose a complex meal. If you're feeling more like taking a nap in the hammock, keep it simple.

4. CONSIDER YOUR OVEN SPACE. How many items that you're doing will need to be in the oven? Will they all need to be in the oven during the last hour? Can some dishes be cooked and kept at room temperature? If the oven space is taken, think of dishes that you can heat on the stove or that don't need heating.

   If you are cooking any quickbread or cake, only make as much batter as your oven can hold. If you need more cake or quickbread than your oven can cook at once, bake in shifts, waiting to make the batter for the second shift until the first set of cakes are cooked. As soon as the wet ingredients are added to the dry, the baking soda or powder are activated, so you can have wet and dry ingredients separately prepared and waiting to be combined.

5. EXPECT A CRISIS. Cooking for large numbers is intense, all-absorbing and can be wildly creative. Don't be surprised if, as the time nears for your guests to arrive, you cook yourself into a frenzy and for a moment you think it's not coming together. It probably

will. That's part of the creative process and what it often takes to get a big meal on the table.

6. MAKE SURE YOU HAVE THE RIGHT EQUIPMENT FOR LARGE NUMBERS. The Hollyhock kitchen has 15 big bins. When we're making salad, we put it immediately into the bin and we know one bin will feed 60 people. Two heaping bins are going to feed 140. We have a mixer that mixes enough dough for 15 loaves of bread, batter for 9 cakes and whips cream for 120 cream puffs.

You probably don't own a comparable piece of equipment, but who does? A big stainless steel bowl can accomplish the same task, it just takes a little more muscle. But think about how many pots, pans and bowls you'll need for the entire process. You may find yourself knocking on a neighbor's door to borrow a few more cake pans. What a great way to build community while making a great meal.

7. MULTIPLY QUANTITIES. Most of the recipes in this book can be simply multiplied to feed a large crowd. Soups are practically foolproof when it comes to expanding numbers. Some breads and pastries won't work this way, however. Be particularly cautious about simply multiplying salt quantities in all recipes. Consult your local chef for guidelines about how much yeast and salt to use when baking bread for large numbers.

8. ENLIST HELP AND HAVE FUN. The Hollyhock kitchen thrives on good conversation, laughter and great music. In order to prepare meals for between 70 and 100 people, Hollyhock needs two cooks, a preparation person and someone just to do the dishes and clean up. Good company, space to work, having people around who are excited about food, and some great music, make it fun to feed large numbers. Get your hands into it. Food feels good.

 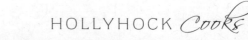

9. PACE YOURSELF. Plan a menu that includes items that can be prepared beforehand. We're always working to deadlines to get the meals on the table. We're seldom late. To keep stress levels down and spirits high, we keep things manageable. We know there's going to be a main dish, a side dish, and sometimes two salads. It's important that we have at least one cold salad done well ahead of time that can chill in the refrigerator. A cold noodle dish can also be done beforehand, as well as bread. That leaves the last minutes for freshly cooked items, entrées and especially seafood. But the trick is to pace the day.

10. ALLOW TIME TO MAKE IT LOOK BEAUTIFUL. Be sure there's adequate opportunity to put out flowers, sprinkle edible blossoms on dishes, and set the table in a visually wonderful way. We all love to eat beautiful food.

11. MAKE THE SPREAD LOOK ABUNDANT. It will seem like you've prepared a feast even if you're short on some dishes. What strikes people first when they come to a meal is the look of the food on the table. After you've laid out the meal, accent the main dishes with bowls of olives, spreads and fresh loaves of bread.

12. IF UNEXPECTED GUESTS SHOW UP, AS THEY OFTEN DO AT HOLLYHOCK, CELEBRATE. Here are a few ways to make it work. Offer an entrée that is portioned in its serving tray, so people aren't tempted to overindulge. Increase the soup by adding whatever vegetables are left in the refrigerator and by putting in more broth. Put on a pot of pasta and place the gourmet entrée at the end of the buffet. That way everyone will fill their plates with the more plentiful items and take delicate portions of what's at the end. Put out smaller plates, if possible. We all fill our plates, whatever their size when the food looks good.

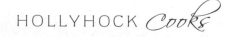

Edible Flowers

DECORATING YOUR FOODS with edible flowers can turn a plain looking meal into a spectacularly beautiful visual feast. Each morning in the Hollyhock kitchen, the gardeners arrive with a basket of freshly picked edible flowers to add beauty to the day's meals. Spring yields tulips, pansies and daylilies. High summer is a bounty of hollyhocks, dahlias and sunflowers. Adding sunny, yellow calendula petals and rich purple borage flowers to a green salad adds bright contrasting colors while remaining mild in taste. Lining a sweet cake or tort with fresh rose petals, lilac or lavender blossoms will add strong floral fragrance and flavor to a dessert. You will be pleasantly surprised to find that many flowers are edible, however not all of them taste good. The following list is of flowers that are both edible and palatable. Unless specified otherwise, use the petals only.

SAVORY HERBS

Basil *(Ocimum basilicum)*

Bee balm *(Monarda didyma)*

Chamomile *(Matricaria recutita)*

Chives *(Allium schoenoprasum)*

Coriander *(Coriandrum sativum)*

Dill *(Anethum graveolens)*

Fennel *(Foeniculum vulgare)*

Garlic chives *(Allium tuberosum)*

Hyssop *(Hyssopus officinalis)*

Lavender *(Lavandula officinalis)*

Lemon balm *(Melissa officinalis)*

Lemon verbena *(Aloysia triphylla)*

Mustard *(Brassica spp.)*

Nasturtium *(Tropaeolum majus)*

Oregano *(Origanum vulgare)*

Rosemary *(Rosmarinus officinalis)*

Saffron crocus *(Crocus sativus)* — Do not confuse with poisonous Fall crocus *(Colshicum autumnale)*

Sage *(Salvia spp.)*

Sweet majorum *(Origanum majorana)*

Sweet woodruff *(Galium odoratum)*

Thyme *(Thymus spp.)*

MILD HERBS

Borage *(Borago officinalis)*

Calendula *(Calendula officinalis)*

Cattail *(Typha latifolia)*

Chickweed *(Stellaria media)*

Chicory *(Chicorium intybus)*

Clover, red *(Trifolium pratense)*

Dandelion *(Taraxacum officinale)*

Elder flower *(Sambucus canadensis or S. caerulea)*

Hawthorn *(Crataegus spp.)*

Hibiscus *(Hibiscus spp.)*

Mallow *(Mallow spp.)*

Mullein *(Verbascum spp.)*

Passionflower *(Passiflora spp.)*

Safflower *(Carthamus tinctorius)* bitter

Salad burnet *(Poterium sanguisorba)*

Yarrow *(Acchillea millefolium)*

Yucca *(Yucca spp.)*

SWEETLY FLORAL

Acacia *(Acacia spp.)*

Apple Blossom *(Malus spp.)*

Carnation or pink *(Dianthus spp.)* Use smaller, fragrant clove pinks
(D. caryophyllus) or cottage pinks *(D. plumarius)*

Columbine *(Aquilegia spp.)*

Day lily *(Hemerocallis spp.)*

Geranium *(Pelargonium spp.)*

Honeysuckle *(Lonicera japonica)*

Jasmine *(Jasminum spp.)* Do not confuse edible jasmine with
poisonous Caroline Jessamine *(Gelsemium sempervirens)*

Lemon blossom *(Citrus limon)*

Lemon Geranium *(Pelagonium crispum)*

Lilac *(Syringa vulgaris)*

Orange blossom *(Citrus sinensis)*

Peppermint geranium *(Pelargonium tomentosum)*

Petunia *(Petunia hybrida)*

Plum blossom *(Prunus domestica)*

Rose *(Rosa spp.)*

Rose geranium *(Pelargonium graveolens)*

Violet *(Viola odorata)*

MILD FLORAL

Bachelor's buttons *(Centaurea)*

Chrysanthemum *(Chrysanthemum morifolium)*

Cowslip *(Primula veris)*

Daisy *(Bellis perennis)*

Dahlias *(Dahlia spp. and cultivars)*

Gladiolus *(Gladiolus spp.)*

Hollyhock *(Alcea rosea)*

Johnny-jump-up *(Viola tricolor)*

Pansy *(Viola wittrockiana)*

Peony *(Paeonica spp.)* — can be bitter

Poppy *(Papaver spp.)* — use only poppy petals

Primrose *(Primula vulgaris)*

Sunflower *(Helianthus annus)*

Squash blossom *(Cucurbita spp.)*

Thistle *(Cirsium spp.)*

Tulip *(Tulipa spp.)*

Viola *(Viola cornuta)*

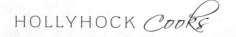

THE AUTHORS AND PHOTOGRAPHER

Moreka Jolar has been cooking at Hollyhock for five years, is passionate about food, and has learned just about everything she knows in the kitchen. She has called Cortes Island her home all her life.

Linda Solomon is an award-winning journalist who has written for *The Los Angeles Times*, *The International Herald Tribune*, *Yoga Journal*, *New Age Journal*, *The Tennessean* and many other publications.

Maria Robledo, originally from Colombia, South America, studied photography at the School of Visual Arts in New York and is noted for her ability to create stunning pictures of ordinary items. She has been the photographer for several cookbooks, including *A New Way to Cook* by Sally Schneider.

THE HOLLYHOCK PRESENTERS

The words of praise for Hollyhock's cooking that appear throughout this book are drawn from the following who present workshops at Hollyhock from time to time:

Margot Anand is the author of several books including *The Art of Everyday Ecstasy*. One of the foremost experts in Western Tantra, she is the founder of six Skydancing Institutes worldwide.

Joan Borysenko is the President of Mind/Body Health Sciences, Inc. in Boulder, Colorado and author of numerous books including *The Woman's Book of Life: The Biology, Psychology and Spirituality of the Feminine Path*.

Tzeporah Berman was a primary architect of the forest markets campaign on Clayoquot Sound. She.is currently the Program Director for Forest Ethics, dedicated to protecting ancient forests, and serves on the Hollyhock Board of Directors.

Sharon Butala is the award-winning author of *The Perfection of the Morning: An Apprenticeship in Nature* and, more recently, *The Garden of Eden*.

Ram Dass, one of the most influential teachers of our time, is author of the 1971 classic *Be Here Now*. His most recent book is *Still Here: Embracing Aging, Changing and Dying*.

Natalie Goldberg is one of North America's best-known writing teachers, and the author of *Writing Down the Bones: Freeing the Writer Within*, and *Wild Mind: Living the Writer's Life*.

Joan Halifax is a Buddhist teacher, anthropologist, and author. A founding member of the Zen Peacemaking Order she is the resident teacher of Upaya Zen Center in Santa Fe, New Mexico.

Andrew Harvey is an internationally renowned poet, novelist, mystical scholar, seeker and spiritual teacher whose bestselling books include *A Journey in Ladakh,* and *One Way of Passion: A Celebration of Rumi*.

Karen Mahon is the Executive Director of the Hollyhock Leadership Institute, a charitable organization that provides training, support and strategy for activists working for a better world.

Ann Mortifee is a singer, songwriter and composer, and past chair of the BC Arts Council. For her contribution to the performing and healing arts, she has been honored with the Order of Canada.

Martin Prechtel was called in 1971 by a Mayan shaman from Guatemala to become his student and to succeed him. He was initiated as a shaman, later becoming a chief initiator and a public leader.

Gregor Robertson, an organic farmer and food activist, is the founder and CEO of Happy Planet Foods, an organic juice company located in BC. He serves on the board of both Hollyhock and the Hollyhock Leadership Institute.

Dr. Andrew Weil is Clinical Professor of Medicine and director of the integrative medicine program at the University of Arizona in Tucson. He is the author of eight books including *Spontaneous Healing, Eating Well for Optimum Health* and *The Healthy Kitchen*.

Acknowledgments

FIRST AND FOREMOST, thank you to those who generously contributed recipes to this project; a percentage of the profit from the sales of this book is going to the Cortes Island Food Bank in your honor. Thanks to everyone who has ever worked in the Hollyhock kitchen and garden. Your dedication and passion for food has made this book possible. We owe a huge debt of gratitude to Debra Fontaine for her wealth of kitchen knowledge and all of her loving support; to Maria Robledo for her taste for beauty; to Nori Fletcher for all the garden goodness she has produced for so many years; to Hanyu Wasyliw and Joy Shipway for their kitchen wisdom; to Martha Abelson, Annie Brae, Rowan Brooks, Annabel Davis, Elena Fraser, Linda Gardner, Chloe Gregg, Carol Newell, Jenica Rayne, Kaeli Robinsong, Shivon Robinsong, Carmen Rosse, Annie Rousseau, David Rousseau, Sylvie Rousseau, Ted Wallbridge, Hanyu Wasyliw, Dianne West, Rosemary Wooldridge, as well as to Debra, Hanyu and Joy for sharing their special recipes; to Patty Manwaring and Rowan Brooks for their typing skills and thoughtful comments; to Diane McIntosh for her cover and page design; to Chris and Judith Plant and the team at New Society Publishers for their commitment to see this project through; and to Heather Wardle for her skilful editing.

Secondly, we'd like to thank each other. Moreka spent endless hours in the kitchen testing every recipe in the book to make sure it came out as deliciously as it sounded on the page. Then she diligently recorded any necessary changes on the recipes, working with Linda to organize them and edit them into the accessible forms you find them in here. Linda interviewed numerous local residents and Hollyhock presenters and staff and incorporated their culinary tales and food philosophy into the book's story of kitchen, garden, island and culture.

Finally, we'd like to thank Dana Bass Solomon, Hollyhock's CEO, for her vision, ideas and constant encouragement. This book would never have happened without her belief that it would.

Beans, fresh
    green, and smoked salmon salad,
        14
    green, Greek salad with feta, 15
    in vegetable korma, 78
    Indian-style, 88
    yellow, with vinaigrette and
        cherry tomatoes, 25
Beet greens, in curried squash, 57
Beets
    in
        borscht, 35
        curried squash, 57
    roasted, with lemon and
        rosemary, 92
Bell peppers. See also Peppers
    hummus with roasted red, 110
    in
        barley pilaf, 91
        chili, 40
        corn soufflé, 178
        cornbread, 124
        enchiladas, 73
        fish stews, 42, 45
        roasted vegetable lasagne, 65
        salads, 15, 16, 18
        sauces, 52, 104
        scrambled tofu, 187
        vegetable curry, 77
        vegetable korma, 78
    stuffed with cherry tomatoes, 83
Berries. See also names of berries
    and apple pie, 151
    banana smoothie, 192
    and melon salad, 186
Biscotti, almond, with fennel and
    black pepper, 150
Biscuits, buttermilk herb, 125
Blackberries
    with honey-lavender custard, 152
    in banana-berry ice, 154
Blending hot liquids, about, 37
Blossom butter, 118
Blueberries
    lemon muffins, 134
    peach, crisp with cardamom, 169
Bok choy, with mushrooms and
    toasted almonds, 81
Borscht, 35

Breads
    about focaccia croutons, 141
    about glazing, freezing, crusts,
doneness, 122, 126, 129, 131, 134
    about puffy pita, 140
    babka with cranberry-almond
        filling, 122
    caraway rye, 126
    French, fennel-topped, 129
    Hollyhock, 131
    honey curry, 132
    zucchini, 148
Breakfast
    applesauce tahini pudding, 176
    black rice pudding with
        banana and lime, 177
    brown rice pudding, maple, 185
    cereal, toasted multigrain and
        seed, 190
    crêpes, whole wheat, 182
    custard with fresh apricots, 179
    eggs, baked, 176
    fruit
        lavender salad, 185
        melon and berry salad, 186
        stewed, 189
    granola, 184
    hash, yam and potato, 187
    muesli with dried cranberries and
        coconut, 186
    oat bake with currants, 189
    oatmeal, 180
    pancakes
        cornmeal buttermilk, 181
        no-wheat, 183
    soufflé, corn, 178
    soy
        hotcakes with orange, 188
        yogurt, 188
    tofu, scrambled, 187
Broccoli, in mixed vegetable salad,
    16
Bulgur wheat, in tabouleh, 27
Buns
    granary, 130
    roulade with green olive
        tapanade, 142
Butter wrappers, about re-using, 136
Buttermilk

    herb biscuits, 125
    in
        cornmeal muffins, 146
        cornmeal pancakes, 181
        oatmeal muffins, 137
        rhubarb coffee cake, 136
    scones, 128
Butters, 116-18
C
Cabbage
    cole slaw
        Asian, 12
        purple cabbage, with
            caraway and currants, 23
Caesar
    tofu
        dip, 106
        dressing, 106
Cakes. See also Coffee cakes
    about slicing, 166
    brownie pudding, 153
    cocoa banana, 159
    gingerbread, 164
    mango ginger upside-down cake,
        168
Cannellini, bean spread with roast-
    ed garlic and sage, 112
Capers
    in eggplant pasta sauce, 52
    salmon salad with chipotle and, 17
Caraway seeds
    purple cabbage slaw with
        currants and, 23
    rye bread, 126
Carrots
    and asparagus sesame stir-fry, 84
    coconut, macaroons, 160
    and fennel roast with fresh dill, 85
    in
        chili, 40
        samosa filling, 48
    in soups
        black bean, 34
        borscht, 35
        lemon-lentil, 46
    in vegetable
        curry, 77
        korma, 78
        salad, 16

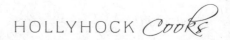

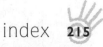

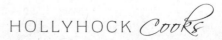

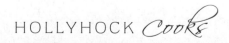

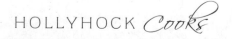

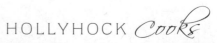
HOLLYHOCK *Cooks*

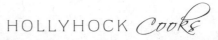

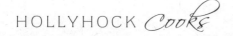

lentil spread with, and curry, 111
Wheat. *See* Whole wheat
Whole wheat
  bagels, 133
  crêpes, 182
  pastry, 123
  scones, 128
Wine, white
  in
    fish stew, 45
    mushroom miso pâté, 112
  mussels in, and Dijon cream, 61
  prawn and snapper stew with
    leeks and, 42

Y
Yams
  in fresh curry paste, 107
  and potato hash, 187
  roasted, with lemon and
    rosemary, 92
  savory, cakes, 67
Yeast dressing, 29
Yogurt
  cardamom sauce, 181
  hazelnut sauce, 90
  in
    green apple raita, 94
    muesli, 186
    salmon mousse quiche, 66
    samosa dough, 48
    shrimp tart, 68
    tzatziki, 95
    vegetable korma, 78
  soy, 188
  spicy squash soup with roasted
    garlic and, 43

Z
Zucchinis
  bread, 148
  in
    chili, 40
    fresh green soup, 39
    roasted vegetable lasagne, 65
    scrambled tofu, 187
    vegetable curry, 77

Index to Chefs

Abelson, Martha
  desserts, 173
  salads and dressings, 20
Brae, Annie
  desserts, 160
Brooks, Rowan
  dips, sauces and pâtés, 103, 107
  entrées, 48
  Side dishes, 93, 99, 100
  soups and stews, 36
Davis, Annabel
  baking, 163
  side dishes, 83
Fontaine, Debra, head chef, 1
  baking, 125, 146
  desserts, 161
  dips, sauces and pâtés, 106, 117
  entrées, 56, 61, 66, 70
Fosker, Stephen
  side dishes, 90
Fraser, Elena
  entrées, 60
Gardner, Linda
  baking, 134, 145, 148
  desserts, 156, 162
  salads and dressings, 13, 14
  soups and stews, 38, 44
Gregg, Chloe
  baking, 135, 138
  dessert, 170
  entrées, 71
Jolar, Moreka
  baking, 122-24, 126-28, 133, 139-
    42, 144, 147
  breakfast, 176-81, 185-90
  desserts, 150-51, 154-55, 157-60,
    164, 168-69
  dips, sauces and pâtés, 102-6, 108-
    16, 118-20
  drinks, 192-93, 195-96
  entrées, 49, 52-53, 55, 58-59, 62-
    65, 67-69, 72-78
  salads and dressings, 12, 14-21,
    23-31
  Side dishes, 80-82, 84-85, 89-95,
    98-100
  soups and stews, 34-35, 37, 40, 42,
    46

Kotilla, Kira
  side dishes, 96-97
Newell, Carol
  entrées, 57
Rayne, Jenica
  dips, sauces and pâtés, 117
  entrées, 50
  side dishes, 87
Robinsong, Kaeli
  soups and stews, 43
Robinsong, Shivon
  breakfast, 176
  desserts, 166
Rosse, Carmen
  baking, 130
  desserts, 152, 165, 167
  entrées, 54
Rousseau, Annie
  salads and dressings, 16
  soups and stews, 38-39
Rousseau, David
  breakfast, 183
  drinks, 196
Rousseau, Sylvie
  breakfast, 182
  salads and dressings, 22
Shipway, Joy
  breakfast, 184
Wallbridge, Ted
  baking, 136
  desserts, 172
Wasyliw, Hanyu
  baking, 129
  breakfast, 181
  desserts, 154, 167, 171
  dips, sauces and pâtés, 105
  entrées, 51
  salads and dressings, 23
  side dishes, 83, 86
  soups and stews, 41, 45
West, Dianne
  baking, 137
  desserts, 153
  side dishes, 98
Wooldridge, Rosemary
  baking, 132
  entrées, 56
  side dishes, 88, 93

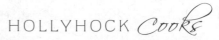

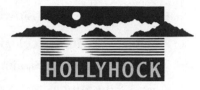

HOLLYHOCK IS A PLACE TO COME TO REPLENISH AND REFOCUS INSIGHT, VISION, AND INTENTIONS. Hundreds of workshops and gatherings for thousands of people and organizations have taken place on this land. It has been the site of communities gathering for shared purpose-a land of immense beauty and magic. On the temperate rainforest coast, the water is sweet. The air is pure. The land, culture, and environs of Hollyhock are so much more untouched than where most of us live our daily lives, yet close enough to reach within a few hours.

HOLLYHOCK EXISTS TO INSPIRE, NOURISH, AND SUPPORT PEOPLE WHO ARE WORKING TO MAKE THE WORLD A BETTER PLACE. Workshops, retreats, conferences, and group bookings provide enriching learning and rejuvenation, supported by dedicated staff on British Columbia's spectacular wilderness coast.

We welcome guests who are learning new life skills, seeking holiday time, participating in an inspiring conference or group meeting, or who are simply wanting to touch in with the natural world, once again. Hollyhock as a place of refuge, a place to dance and sing, a place to shift thinking and perception, a place to have a great conversation, or as a place to simply enjoy the magic of being quiet.

For more information: 800-933-6339, www.hollyhock.ca

If you have enjoyed *Hollyhock Cooks,* you might also enjoy other

BOOKS TO BUILD A NEW SOCIETY

Our books provide positive solutions for people who want to make a difference. We specialize in:

**Sustainable Living • Ecological Design and Planning • Natural Building & Appropriate Technology
New Forestry • Environment and Justice • Conscientious Commerce • Progressive Leadership
Educational and Parenting Resources • Resistance and Community • Nonviolence**

For a full list of NSP's titles, please call 1-800-567-6772 or check out our web site at:
www.newsociety.com

New Society Publishers

ENVIRONMENTAL BENEFITS STATEMENT

New Society Publishers has chosen to produce this book on New Leaf EcoBook 100, recycled paper made with 100% post consumer waste, processed chlorine free, and old growth free.

For every 5,000 books printed, New Society saves the following resources:[1]

40	Trees
3,587	Pounds of Solid Waste
3,947	Gallons of Water
5,148	Kilowatt Hours of Electricity
6,521	Pounds of Greenhouse Gases
28	Pounds of HAPs, VOCs, and AOX Combined
10	Cubic Yards of Landfill Space

[1]Environmental benefits are calculated based on research done by the Environmental Defense Fund and other members of the Paper Task Force who study the environmental impacts of the paper industry.

For more information on this environmental benefits statement, or to inquire about environmentally friendly papers, please contact New Leaf Paper – info@newleafpaper.com Tel: 888 • 989 • 5323.

NEW SOCIETY PUBLISHERS